Family Policy

Family Policy

Fran Wasoff and Ian Dey

Routledge
Taylor & Francis Group
LONDON AND NEW YORK

Routledge,
2 Park Square, Milton Park, Abingdon, Oxon, OX14 4RN
711 Third Avenue, New York, NY 10017, USA

First issued in hardback 2017

Routledge is an imprint of the Taylor & Francis Group, an informa business

First Published 2000 by Routledge

Cover Design: Clare Truscott
Cover Illustration: Tom Saecker/The Organisation
Typeset by Central Southern Typesetters, Eastbourne, East Sussex

ISBN 13: 978-1-138-41142-5 (hbk)
ISBN 13: 978-0-9533571-5-4 (pbk)

Contents

Tables

Figures

Acknowledgements

Our thanks to Pete Alcock for suggesting that we write this book, to our colleagues in the Department of Social Policy at The University of Edinburgh and The School of Social Service Administration at the University of Chicago for their support, to our reviewers for their careful and constructive comments, and to Pat McNeill at Gildredge Press for his patience in awaiting its completion. Our greatest debt as always is to our families for their faith and forbearance during its production.

The order in which the authors are listed was decided by the toss of a coin.

Series introduction

Social policy in the United Kingdom has undergone major changes since the mid-1970s and particularly since the election of the Thatcher government in 1979. The post-war consensus is long gone and far-reaching changes have been made in every area of social policy. These changes, of principle and of practice, have been guided both by ideology and by the context of a post-industrial and increasingly globalized economy. The emergence of New Labour has added a new and still developing dimension of change.

The growing number of students of social policy, in higher education, on advanced level course such as AS/A levels and GNVQs, and training for professional qualifications, have to make sense of this fast-changing scene, to consider the long-term effects, and to make their own judgements of the deep-rooted issues of value that are involved.

This new series of introductory textbooks is aimed specifically at these students. The books are not academic monographs but short, tightly-structured texts written with both the academic student and the trainee professional in mind. All the authors are currently involved in teaching and in policy development.

The books are designed to be aids to learning. Each book includes a brief history and background to its policy area, a review of current provision, and a discussion of future issues and possible developments. They thus present students with a concise, clear and up-to-date summary of what they need to know and understand in each area of social policy.

Family policy: definitions, values and aims

1

Outline
What is family policy? In this chapter, we look at efforts to define family policy in terms of its aims and effects. Our approach involves identifying the main activities we associate with families, and considering how and why society takes in interest in these activities. We consider the different approaches that can be taken to analysing policy, and note the importance of social policy focusing on needs, problems and rights. Different perspectives on family policy are identified through the on-going debate about 'family values'. We contrast libertarian and interventionist values, although conflicts over the role of the state in family policy (that is, over 'means') are overlaid by differences in the ends – traditionalist, egalitarian and pragmatist – that the various protagonists pursue.

FAMILIES

> The family is the bedrock of a decent, civilised and stable society
> (DSS 1998d, p. 13)

Humans are 'family animals' (Tudge 1995, p. 214). We are born into families, we create families, we live in families and we are buried by families. Families provide the basic social geography through which we negotiate our paths through life. They form the basic fabric of social intercourse. For Europeans surveyed in 1993, the family remained their most important social value (Hantrais and Letablier 1996, p. 65).

Exceptions tend to prove the rule. Utopian visions of abolishing the family are hard to realize. Experiments in living in alternative social groups often underline the resilience of family forms (Robertson 1991). Even in the most famous case, the kibbutz, it is claimed that people have 'returned to the stereotype' (Ridley 1994, pp. 251–2).

WHAT IS A FAMILY?

Families are familiar, but also elusive. They change according to context. Who is invited to the wedding? To the funeral? To the family meal? Who gives and who inherits? Who raises the children, and who cares for ageing parents? We count ourselves as 'family' for some purposes, but not for others. We 'belong' (an archaic but revealing expression) to several families – the nuclear family, the extended family, the ancestral family – which form multiple and overlapping sets. Family boundaries are hard to draw.

This dual character of families – familiar yet elusive – offers a fractured foundation for 'family policy'. On one side, we have the simple and appealing image of the ideal family – hailed as a haven of human happiness. On the other, there are the complex realities of family life, with its dark secrets of conflict, exploitation and abuse.

Definitions of families vary across countries and within countries, for different purposes. Some of the problems of defining families are evident in gathering statistics. We may distinguish families (people who are related but may not live together) from households (people who live together but may not be related). However, living arrangements and relationships are often complex. Do we regard everyone under one roof (sharing the same facilities) as a 'family', or only those recognized as related, such as partners and their 'dependent' children? A young person living with their parents might be included or excluded by different definitions. At what age and in what circumstances do children cease to count as members of their birth family, rather than as adults and independent families in their own right? In some European countries, 18 is the limit; in others, no limit is applied. Should partnership refer only to married couples or also include those in 'consensual unions' (living together as if married)? Should partnership refer only to heterosexual couples, or (as in the next census in Britain) also recognize same-sex couples?

WHAT IS FAMILY POLICY?

'Family policy' too is a strange phrase, marrying terms that often have little connection. There is no consensus over what family policy is or ought to be. Family policy can be narrowly focused or broad brush; its aims can be explicit or implicit; and in orientation it can be minimalist or maximalist, or somewhere in between. Family policy can be comprehensive or selective in approach; it can be coherent, or unco-ordinated across different policy areas. It can involve policies for all families or only for some. Not surprisingly, different writers place the boundaries of family policy in different places.

Explicit family policy

At one end of the spectrum, we could consider only those policies deliberately addressing family issues: a narrow, focused definition of family policy.

> Social policy is generally described as family policy when the family is the deliberate target of specific actions, and the measures initiated are designed to have an impact on family resources and, ultimately, on family structure
>
> (Hantrais 1999, p. 104)

This is similar to the definition of explicit family policy by Kamerman and Kahn (1978, p. 3):

> specific programs and policies designed to achieve specified, explicit goals regarding the family; [or] programs and policies which deliberately do things to and for the family, but for which there are no agreed-upon overall goals regarding the family

Policies relating to childcare and income maintenance, including child benefit, and the law regulating parental obligations to children would normally fall within this definition. Recent government policies (such as the National Childcare Strategy and the Working Families Tax Credit) can be seen as explicit family policies.

Proposals may sometimes be presented as explicit 'family policy' for easier consumption, even though their real concern lies elsewhere – such as reducing public expenditure or increasing employment. For example, the Child Support Act is widely regarded as a measure to reduce public expenditure, despite more publicized aims of increasing paternal responsibility and improving procedures for determining maintenance.

Implicit family policy

At the other end of the spectrum, we could include policies with other objectives that have consequences for family life. Kamerman and Kahn identify implicit family policy as 'government actions and policies not specifically or primarily addressed to the family, but which have indirect consequences' (1978, p. 3).

The family is then one context within which social policies operate. This defines 'family policy' in terms of effects, as 'everything that government does to and for the family' (Kamerman and Kahn 1978, p. 3). For even where 'family' and 'policy' are apparently unconnected, it need not mean that one does not affect the other. Indirect family policies include many housing policies, health policies, education and employment policies, criminal policies and so on. Indeed it is difficult to think of social policies that do not have consequences for at least some families. This would be even more evident if, as some critics advocate, governments were to introduce 'family impact statements' to predict the effects that policies pursued for other purposes might have on families.

National family policy

Family policy can also describe an overall approach by government to the family – whether or not a state has a specific focus on 'the family' in its activities, and how 'the family' features in the policy process. In some countries, the family is seen as a core social institution for which the state bears responsibility, whereas others consider the family a private domain in which the state should not interfere. The extent to which family policy is institutionalized in the constitution and structures of government depends on its traditions as well as upon how it views state intervention in family life. Some countries have a Minister for the Family. In others, family policies range across a number of areas of government activity.

Britain is conventionally thought not to have a national family policy at all. Policy is initiated by parliament and modified by law and practice without a constitutional framework setting out rights and establishing obligations. In practice, policies develop within policy 'arenas' in which government departments loom large, although other agencies such as professional organizations, employers, and service deliverers may also be key players. Families themselves may be poorly represented within this arena, although the rise of research foundations, think-tanks and pressure groups has had some impact in extending the terms and tone of debate. In particular the issues of child poverty and child abuse have focused attention on the needs and rights of children. These have been reinforced by the active role of the European Court of Human Rights, and the Labour government elected in

1997 is due to implement the Human Rights Act (1998) in the first year of the new millennium. In the meantime, the Labour government has created a Ministerial Group on the Family, headed by Jack Straw, the Home Secretary. Its discussion document *Supporting Families* (Home Office/Ministerial Group on the Family 1998) maps an overall approach to family issues across a number of ministerial briefs. It remains to be seen if this signals the beginning of a national family policy for the UK.

Whether in terms of purposes or effects, it is difficult to disentangle family issues from a wider policy agenda. Given this complexity, it is probably unwise to seek a simple definition of family policy. Take the claim that 'the objective of family policy is to redistribute resources so as to eliminate differences in the standards of living for households with and without children' (Hantrais and Letablier 1996, p. 149). We may sympathize with this objective. But it is not one which recent British governments have pursued with any vigour, since the income gap between families with and without children has widened over the post-war years. Whether and how families and policies are connected in this or any other way remains an open question. We can consider how 'families' and 'policies' interact, without presuming that policies have an intended impact on family life and family structure. These interactions may be clarified if we consider what families do – and why the wider society takes an interest in these activities.

WHAT DO FAMILIES DO?

There are some activities we can readily identify with family life:

- reproduction
- socialization
- care and protection
- distribution
- work.

These have all become a focus of concern for social policy in recent years.

Reproduction

Humans reproduce through families. We do not all have children – but we are all born of at least one parent. As we all have a stake in the reproduction of the next generation, societies may try to influence reproductive activity. At one extreme, China has limited families to one child. This policy has produced an unintendedly high male-female ratio (as high as 28 : 1 in some parts of the country) – reflecting the covert use of infanticide to realize a widespread preference for male over female children. Other countries (e.g. France) have tried to stimulate rather than limit births, although using incentives rather than regulation.

More typically, policies reflect or reinforce cultural assumptions about who should form families, who is 'fit' to reproduce and who should bear the costs of reproduction. Two factors have combined to push these issues to centre stage:

- Social change – with a growth in divorce, cohabitation, and re-marriage; a trend towards later marriage and childbirth; and a rise in extra-marital births and childlessness.
- Technological change – with new methods of reproduction challenging 'natural' (cultural) preconceptions about how children are and ought to be conceived. Artificial control over reproduction allows selection by sex, disability or (the most popular criterion in selecting eggs) intelligence – posing the problem of whether and how this should be socially regulated.

Controversies over teenage mothers, lone parents and same-sex or same-race adoption are raised as society tries to adjust to – or resist – the implications of change.

Socialization

Having borne children, someone has to raise them, and typically this is done in families. Families remain the main medium through which a baby becomes an adult. Nowadays, however, families share this activity with other institutions and occupations, notably schools, nurseries and childminders. Societies too have a stake in the process and outcomes of socialization. Educational, childcare and other policies try to ensure that youngsters crossing from childhood to adulthood make it successfully to the other side.

Issues of socialization have become more pressing as societies adjust to a more integrated and competitive global economy by emphasizing education and skills as a route to greater competitiveness. Youth unemployment and rising crime rates have sharpened this concern. Arguments about the emergence of a youth 'underclass' (Murray *et al.* 1990; MacDonald 1997) have focused attention on the role of the family in effective socialization. The racial overtones of this debate in Britain have been muted (at least compared with America) but they are significant nonetheless. British concern for socialization has centred on the negative consequences for children of family 'disruption' and 'breakdown' (both, note, very value-laden terms).

Care and protection

Families are often contrasted with the marketplace, because families are formed (it is assumed) mainly through emotional rather than economic bonds, expressing intimate rather than instrumental relationships. Whatever its validity, this contrast directs attention to the caring activities and the protection associated with family life. People in families tend to care for and protect each other, not just in illness or infirmity but through everyday activities promoting psychological and physical well-being. And society has a stake in that caring process, not least because it may have to step into the breach if care breaks down.

Issues of care centre on what care should be provided at home, and by whom. These have become more pressing with the shift from institutional to community care, and a corresponding emphasis on the role and contribution of family members in providing care. Feminists have emphasized the gender implications of shifting care from institutions to families. While on one hand the government looks to women to provide unpaid informal care, on the other it encourages them to take up formal paid employment. More generally, policies to increase the choice of services and to encourage independent living raise questions about the provision and control of care resources, and how far families receive effective support for caring activities.

Recognition that child abuse is a widespread phenomenon has tended to undermine the traditional view of parenting as a private preserve, justify the intervention of the state in family life, and encourage the development of greater recognition of children's rights. Feminists have emphasized that there is also a need for the protection of adults from violence within families.

Resource distribution

Families are arenas where resources are distributed. Assumptions about property transfer between generations were a defining feature of family form – for example, promoting inheritance by the first male son in defiance of the logic of genetics (Jones 1993).

Today we worry less about inheritance, and more about the transfer of resources within the current generation. 'Who gets what?' is now a question asked about the family meal and not just the family silver. Policy can affect the answer, not least in influencing the opportunities provided for family members to acquire independent resources. And society may be concerned with the outcome, if only because failure to transfer resources may mean that some family members rely on state support.

Resource issues often focus on family income. Budgets are followed by analyses of how tax and benefit measures may affect the income of different types of family – whether and which families will be 'better off' or 'worse off'. Such assessments consider questions of equity (how do families with children fare compared to those without, for example) and adequacy (whether families are going to have enough to live on). Both equity and adequacy have traditionally been judged by comparing families in different circumstances, but in recent years attention has focused on distribution within families as well as between them. One issue here is whether women are at higher risk of poverty within the family because of their more limited access to independent income.

Work

In our acquisitive society, it has become fashionable to see the family as an institution through which goods and services are purchased and consumed. We tend to regard production of these goods and services as a labour market activity outside a family setting. But work remains a vital family activity, required both to generate resources (through paid employment) and to sustain everyday life (through unpaid labour in the household). Here the question is not 'Who gets what?' but 'Who does what?'. Society has a stake in the outcome, not least because both family and labour market are affected if paid and unpaid work are out of balance.

Work issues often focus on how women might be released from household work to take up employment in the labour market. Policies have tried to improve childcare provision and incentives to take paid employment. However, women's participation in the labour market still stirs controversy over how well they can fulfil their domestic roles. The traditional division of labour within the family has been challenged, notably by feminists, but measures to encourage 'new men' to undertake a fairer share of domestic labour have still to make a serious impact on the policy agenda (or indeed on family life).

These, then, are some of the family activities which, for better or worse, policies seek to influence, or indirectly or inadvertently affect. These activities provide the framework around which this book is structured.

ANALYSING FAMILY POLICIES

As well as considering what families do, we also need to consider what family policy does, and how it can analysed. Zimmerman (1995, p. 12) identifies a range of activities (or functions) associated with family policies, including policies to:

- distribute or redistribute resources
- regulate behaviour
- create or modify procedures and structures.

These activities are evident in programmes such as Child Benefit, in efforts to reduce conflict during divorce, or to create support for those providing informal care. Zimmerman (1995, p. 7) also identifies a range of conceptual frameworks through which family policy can be analysed, including analysis of policy as:

- an outcome of rational or incremental choices
- a reflection of elite or cultural preferences
- a product of institutional structures and processes
- a result of competition between contending interest groups.

These frameworks are not mutually exclusive, and although in this book we focus on the role of governments in choosing among family policy options, the influence of institutional structures, interest groups and ideologies in shaping policy can be readily identified in various policy fields. For example, the structure of the social security system is important in shaping redistributive policies; potentially conflicting interests influence policies in areas like child protection and informal care; and ideological preferences have a marked impact (as we shall see) on how family structures and activities are perceived and evaluated.

Family policy and social policy

Zimmerman tends to identify family policy with social policy in general, with social policy being seen as a means of stabilizing and supporting families whose needs cannot be met by the market. However, it is possible to distinguish social policies which have other ends and means. For example, educational policies may be important instruments for fostering cultural development or economic competitiveness. Health services may have a vital role in maintaining the productive efficiency of the working population. Social security programmes may be concerned with maintaining or enforcing work incentives. In this book, we focus more on policies which are concerned primarily with influencing family activities, rather than these wider social policy agendas.

Nevertheless, social policy does identify some general discourses through which to consider the evolution of family policies. There are three in particular which it may be useful to identify here:

- The first concerns whether and how family policies are oriented to meeting the *needs* of families. For example, we might ask whether Income Support provides an adequate standard of living for those families who depend upon it. Recognizing needs tends to imply a moral imperative to satisfy them.
- The second concerns the ways in which family activities are defined as *problems*, and how these problems are to be managed if not resolved. For example, we might ask whether violence (including 'smacking' a child) within the family is a problem, and if so what should be done about it. A social problems perspective tends to provoke interventionist measures aimed at changing attitudes or controlling behaviour.
- The third concerns the role of *rights*, most notably in identifying appropriate or inappropriate forms of intervention in family affairs. For example, there has been a shift towards recognizing the rights of children, both to have their interests taken into account and their voice heard in decisions which affect them – at least in the context of child protection policies. A rights perspective tends to raise questions of fairness and equity, although as rights are enforced at someone else's expense, they also raise issues of the cost and constraint on liberty involved in recognizing them. The increased prominence of 'human rights' in recent years has also been matched by a growing emphasis on the duties and responsibilities of citizenship.

Policies may differ significantly in their aims and means, according to whether they give priority to meeting needs, managing problems or recognizing rights. For example, in the 1970s policy focused on the needs of lone-parent families, and additional benefits and premiums were introduced to meet those needs. In the 1990s, policy has focused on the problems posed by lone parents, notably the problems of dependency and the cost to the taxpayer, and measures have been taken to reduce their benefits and make entitlement conditional on attending interviews about returning to work.

These distinctive but overlapping discourses have a powerful impact on family policies, and any particular policy agenda – such as support for informal care in the community – is likely to be influenced in different ways by each of them. Thus the rights of disabled or frail older people to live as normal a family life as possible have influenced community care policies; the problems of reconciling caring and careers has provoked a raft of 'family-friendly' policies, while the needs of informal carers have been subject of a recent government initiative.

THE DEBATE OVER FAMILY VALUES

Society is trying to come to terms with changes in family roles and relationships. Should it encourage a fairer division of domestic labour, or should this be a private concern? Should cohabiting couples be treated in the same way as married couples? Should fertility treatment or adoption be made available to same-sex couples? Should the state try to influence how families socialize their children, for example in relation to homework? Should non-resident fathers be held responsible for child support? Should parents be held responsible for the socially unacceptable behaviour of their children? These questions tend to reflect moral concerns arising from change in traditional normative frameworks, but are often sharpened by anxiety and arguments over the financial and social costs of coping with change. It is not always easy to distinguish issues of principle (what should be the responsibilities of non-resident parents?) from pragmatic concerns (such as reducing the cost of state support for lone parents).

'The family' has become the subject of fierce political debate about deeply held social and moral values. By the mid-1990s, there seemed a sense of crisis over 'the family', provoking a widespread debate over 'family values'. This debate emphasized the family as a problem for society, with little reference to either needs or rights. The problem that most exercised politicians concerned family breakdown and the growth of lone-parent families – with a tendency to blame the social ills associated with youth (as in the murder of James Bulger by two young boys) with failures in family socialization. Another prominent issue concerned the family's capacity to care for its older members, especially given the presumed decline in the extended family, the shift to community care, the growth of women's participation in the labour market, and the supposed 'burden' of an ageing population. It is ironic that some obvious 'solutions' to the latter problem – such as immigration – are excluded from the political agenda.

Is the family in crisis?

Because it commands attention (and captures headlines) this is a common cry. It implies that there is something fundamental and perhaps fatally wrong with the family, which only moral courage and decisive action will put right. But what exactly is the problem? Those who claim there is a crisis in family life point to the erosion of family values leading to moral and social disintegration, most evident in the unhappy consequences of family 'breakdown':

> It is becoming increasingly clear to all but the most blinkered of social scientists that the disintegration of the nuclear family is the principal source of so much misery and unrest
>
> (*Sunday Times* editorial cited by Roseneil and Mann in Silva 1996, p. 199)

Social change has raised fears that families are failing to carry out their various activities (reproduction, socialization, care, work and distribution) in ways acceptable to society.

A key issue for critics is that of moral responsibility – both to children and to society. The journalist Melanie Phillips sees divorce as symptomatic of adults behaving irresponsibly, seeking 'fun' and abandoning marriages simply because they are less than perfect. British parents are less likely than their European counterparts to see 'bringing up and educating children' as the most important family role and more likely to see the family's role as 'to provide love and affection' (Pugh *et al.* 1994, p. 11). They prefer personal satisfactions through companionate relationships rather than through fulfilling formal roles and responsibilities – such as the socialization of children.

Figure 1.1 Companionate marriage

A positive slant on 'companionate' marriage is offered by Janet Reibsten, who suggests the following as key to a happy and enduring marriage:

- Protection – treating each other with delicacy and a welcoming degree of co-reliance.
- Focus – giving attention, time and energy to each other.
- Gratitude – demonstrating appreciation and acknowledging your partner's value to you.
- Balance – mutual give and take.
- Pleasure – enjoying your marriage and delighting in each other.

For Reibsten, successful marriages are based on 'protective love' and mutual interdependence – relating to the quality of personal relationships rather than any notion of duty. (Cited by Cohen 1997.)

The 'misery' of family breakdown includes poorer health and educational progress, greater risks of drug-taking and early pregnancy, and higher rates of delinquency and crime among its victims. Problems of indiscipline, drugs and crime are attributed to failures of parenting. The issue of 'absent' fathers is a prominent theme, taken as a key factor in explaining subsequent delinquency and crime. But there are also concerns over 'absent' mothers – whose participation in employment prevents them spending adequate time with their children. This theme is much loved by the media and politicians, for whom unmarried teenage mothers have also proved an irresistible target. They have often been accused of using pregnancy for selfish ends, to obtain benefit and jump the housing queue.

Matching the accusation of an abrogation of parental responsibility, critics like Phillips argue, is a broader irresponsibility to society. In the absence of a breadwinner, the taxpayer often picks up the bill. One estimate suggests that family breakdown costs the country more than £4 billion a year in benefits, lost tax, and legal and health bills (Dobson and Moyes 1996). Thus private satisfactions are maximized through irresponsible attitudes, at public cost. These twin concerns have been merged most effectively in the 'underclass' thesis, where illegitimacy, unemployment and crime (the main characteristics associated with the 'underclass') are seen as tied together in an unholy mess of disreputable behaviours indulged at society's expense (Murray 1994).

By emphasizing the role of the state in creating conditions conducive to social immorality, the underclass thesis also puts the family and its failings in the spotlight. This has stimulated policies aimed at making parents more responsible. The 1990s opened with child support legislation to impose obligations on 'absent' fathers. It continued with a hotly-contested review of divorce legislation introducing (and subsequently abandoning) a 'cooling off' period and mediation as a prelude to divorce. The benefit premiums that recognized the extra costs of lone parenthood were frozen and later abolished. The courts were given powers to fine parents for the delinquent behaviour of their children. Government can now impose curfews on children, insist on courses in parenting for the parents of young offenders, and insist on children completing set periods of homework.

Responses to the 'moral backlash'

While those concerned with moral disintegration and social pathology have dominated the debate over 'family values', they have yet to convince their critics. There are at least four responses to the 'moral backlash':

- historical
- philosophical
- social
- political.

The historical response

The historical response is that we have been here many times before. Take the complaint in an Egyptian inscription 6,000 years ago: 'Our earth is degenerate. Children no longer obey their parents'. Or take Aristophanes in the fifth century BC, already nostalgic for the 'good old days, when children ... were seen not heard, led a simple life, in short, were well brought up'. There is nothing particularly 'current' about issues such as cohabitation. Family problems are not new but have merely seemed more pressing because family life became unusually conformist and stable in the previous half century. Even that period of stability (or conformity) may have been more myth than substance. It was in the 1950s that words like 'teenager' and 'delinquent' acquired common currency, and youthful 'rebellion' was constructed as a social problem. Such problems are 'discovered' anew (and as new) by each passing (and ageing) generation – although they have perhaps acquired a particular piquancy as the millennium approaches.

The philosophical response

The philosophical response challenges the premise that society is in a state of moral decline. It argues that the transition from deferential attitudes, authoritarian institutions and ascribed social roles has led, if anything, to a remoralization of society. Choice rather than unthinking obedience is the hallmark of a moral order, so 'we now live in a more demanding moral climate' (Jacques 1996). Moral issues may have become messier, in that they cannot be resolved by simple rules (or dogmas) prescribed by Church and State. Moreover, technological change confronts us with new choices and uncertainties – such as cloning – which cannot easily be resolved in terms of traditional authority. As this has given way to more democratic forms, the range of moral concerns has broadened and individual morality has deepened. Arguably, the soap opera has become the moral laboratory of our time, where stories explore complex personal dilemmas without presuming a uniform moral code.

The social response

The social response challenges any simple equation of family problems with family pathologies. Discussing the outcomes of divorce, for example, Utting notes that a 'formidable body of research ... links adverse social conditions to the chances that children will fail to thrive'; so 'while individual responsibility is relevant, a more balanced discussion needs to take account of the indirect and external influences' (Utting 1995, p. 32). Utting cites the rise in poverty and inequality, and its adverse effects on child health and educational performance. The problem is less family 'breakdown' as such, than the increasingly adverse social and economic effects that it can precipitate. Moral issues need to be considered within a changing social context.

The political response

The political response suggests the moral backlash is itself 'pathological', distorting social realities and producing inadequate and often counter-productive policies (Phoenix 1996). The moral backlash serves a political purpose, critics suggest, in 'blaming the victim' and so legitimating policies designed to reduce welfare spending at their expense (Roseneil and Mann 1996). Thus the moral agenda serves as a thinly disguised tool for reducing state welfare – although this agenda is hard to sustain when governments are embarrassed by the moral 'transgressions' of their own members.

THE ROLE OF THE STATE IN FAMILY LIFE

The 'family values' debate has been fuelled by the clash between traditional moralists and their critics. Any debate over 'the family' soon becomes a debate over the state, and what role if any it should play in regulating family affairs.

As the boundaries between state and family 'are often confused and contested, with ambiguous areas of responsibility' (Harding 1996, p. 177) there is ample scope for conflict over state intervention in family life. To clarify the debate, Harding contrasts two extreme positions. The first is an authoritarian position, in which the state has clearly defined and rigidly enforced objectives for families. This is contrasted with a libertarian, minimalist or laissez-faire perspective, in which the family is regarded as a private arena beyond state concern.

The authoritarian approach aims to enforce certain behaviours and prohibit others – policies to raise or lower fertility rates and hence population growth being a common example. The state regulates through law but may also try to inculcate moral values through education and media propaganda. There is often a close connection between secular and religious authority, shaping attitudes to issues like contraception, abortion and divorce. More generally, an interventionist perspective has faith in the role of state in affecting family life, for example policies to introduce parental control or responsibility orders, allowing parents of 'delinquents' to be fined, tagged or trained in their parental role.

The libertarian approach, by contrast, has a policy of 'no policy'. It holds that in principle, there should be no legal regulation of marriage or parenthood and no prescription regarding sexual/reproductive behaviour, or patterns of living and mutual support. The state should treat people in their private lives only as individuals. From this perspective, the state has no moral authority to regulate parenting. Its own record in 'parenting' children, libertarians argue, hardly establishes its credibility in this regard (consider the series of child abuse scandals in residential homes). Nor is it clear, they suggest, what model of 'parenting' is to be imposed. Fashions in child-rearing change quickly and there is little agreement on how to do it.

As 'ideal models' these authoritarian and libertarian perspectives illuminate conflicts of principle but may be a poor guide to the positions taken up in practice. Between these extremes, Harding recognizes a continuum of positions, depending partly on forms of enforcement – through regulation, incentives or the force of tacit assumptions. These also reflect the extent to which family policy is proactive (pursuing its own agenda) or reactive (responding to problems only as they arise). The more one leans toward proactive regulation, the more interventionist the perspective.

However, we tend to see such intervention as legitimate when we approve its aims and illegitimate when we do not. Although views differ over the scope for state intervention in family life, we cannot separate conflict over means from the different agendas which people pursue.

Competing agendas

To compare these different agendas, we shall adapt a classification which distinguishes between traditionalist, egalitarian and pragmatic perspectives (cf. Millar 1998, p. 123).

The traditionalist perspective

The traditionalists are major defenders of 'the family' as an institution. Craven *et al.* (1982) suggest that the traditional family tends to be seen variously as:

- *A bulwark of freedom* – a countervailing force to the encroaching powers of state and bureaucracy.
- *A seat of authority* – especially paternal authority, which fosters stability and effective socialization to counter-balance the social disorganization arising with the industrialization and urbanization of modern life.
- *A source of community* – of personal intimacy and social cohesion, but rooted in social roles and obligations rather than individual rights.
- *A means of reproduction* – of the workers, citizens and entrepreneurs on whom the future of society (or 'the nation') depends.

Traditionalists see the traditional family as a key institution for maintaining social order as well as the procreator of future generations. Morgan (1998, p. 71), for example, stresses the importance of marriage as the context for child-rearing, asking if married couples are an endangered species:

> Marriage is an age-old and universal framework for the ordering and understanding of family organisation, parental perspectives and behaviour, which creates obligations between adult parties, their kin, and the couple and their children. ... What we are witnessing now is not the formalisation of other 'family structures', but the de-regulation of the conjugal nuclear family which we have known for centuries.
>
> (Morgan 1998, p. 71)

In policy terms, this involves privileging or restoring marriage as a particular family form.

The egalitarian perspective

In egalitarian perspectives, 'the family' is assessed in more ambivalent terms, both valued as a counterpoint to market forces and criticized as a means of reproducing social inequalities. Egalitarian perspectives encompass a range of different approaches, depending on whether the emphasis is placed on such social divisions as class, gender, ethnicity, disability or sexual orientation.

With regard to class inequalities, the egalitarian agenda has been concerned with the family's role in reproducing class inequalities between families. Through inheritance, and through privileged access to goods and services such as education, housing and health, some children gain advantage at the expense of others. This leads to concern with the conditions which marginalize or exclude families from participating fully in society. Thus the job of government can be seen as 'to make sure that families can meet the needs of children, and to step in where they cannot' (Coote 1995).

The feminist agenda has focused on inequalities within families and how family responsibilities contribute to gender inequality in the public sphere. The family is seen as 'a pivot of oppressive socialisation' (Craven *et al.* 1982, p. 20) trapping women in limited roles established through marriage, the sexual division of labour and unequal distribution of resources within the family. Instead of restoring traditional roles, it is argued that policies should support and encourage change:

> If families are to be strengthened, we need to redefine the roles and responsibilities of men and women. Both should have a chance to be loving and attentive parents ... as well as breadwinners
> (Coote 1995)

From this perspective, arguments are advanced to protect children growing up in families and give legitimacy to new family patterns, which no longer privilege marriage or heterosexual relationships.

Concerns with ethnicity focus mainly on inequalities between families. Cultural stereotypes about family obligations and roles vary according to ethnic group, leading to different and potentially misleading assumptions, for example about the extent of support for family members among minorities. Such stereotypes can affect access to services, notably in health, education, and social security. Differences in family patterns across ethnic groups also render some more vulnerable to reductions in state welfare, such as the recent cuts in lone-parent benefits. However, the 'racial' dimension of political campaigns such as those against lone parents is rarely made explicit. This is also the case with immigration and asylum, where the state itself can disrupt and divide families, and deny them minimum living standards, as part of its attempt to prevent 'undesirable' migration.

The egalitarian perspective also raises important questions for family policy regarding disability and sexual orientation. Both the disability and the gay and lesbian movements have pressed for equal rights with regard to reproduction and family formation. This includes rights to marry, conceive, adopt children, and live a 'normal' family life.

The pragmatic perspective

Finally, there is a more pragmatic and reformist tradition, which sees some merit in accepting and adapting to changes in family life and trying to use family policies both to promote their positive aspects and to mitigate their worst consequences. The pragmatist position is illustrated in the IPPR publication, *The Family Way*, in which Coote, Harman and Hewitt (1998, p. 113) argue that:

> [Family] policies should be adaptable, to support all kinds of family. In these changing times, fewer families conform to the traditional model of family life – and we know that this trend is likely to increase. Public policy should therefore seek to support the process of family life, whatever the shape or size of the family unit.

Pragmatists doubt the state's capacity to regulate behaviour (such as divorce) in defiance of the social and economic circumstances which shape it.

National policy

The clash between these perspectives was evident in the controversies over the reform of divorce in England and Wales in 1995. Traditionalists viewed the legislation as undermining of marriage, by making divorce easier and by extending protection from domestic violence to cohabitees. Egalitarians and pragmatists saw it as an opportunity to reduce conflict on divorce and as some recognition of greater diversity in family composition.

While it is possible to differentiate political perspectives in a broad way, it is less obvious how to categorize the policies of particular states or parties. Nevertheless Gauthier (1996) classifies the family policies of different countries into four types:

- Pro-natalist family policies primarily concerned with maintaining or increasing fertility, e.g. France.
- Pro-traditional family policies concerned with supporting traditional family roles and functions, e.g. Germany.
- Pro-egalitarian family policies concerned with promoting and supporting gender equality in family life, e.g. Sweden, Denmark.
- Pro-family but selectively interventionist only for families with identified needs, but otherwise non-interventionist, e.g. USA, UK.

If we regard natalist policies (both pro-natal and anti-natal) as one variant of the traditional perspective, Gauthier's typology parallels quite closely the distinctions we have drawn between traditional, egalitarian and pragmatist perspectives, with the UK in her view tending to fall into the latter camp.

When compared with other European countries with a tradition of state intervention in family life, the UK is often classified as a strong advocate of the family as a private domain (Hantrais and Letablier 1996, p. 143). However, the Labour government elected in 1997 espouses a pragmatist approach, combining elements of both egalitarian and traditionalist perspectives. It recognizes that 'what families – all families – have a right to expect from government is support' and that it 'is not for the state to decide whether people marry or stay together.'

(Home Office/ Ministerial Group on the Family 1998, p. 2 and p. 30). It also states that:

> ... marriage is still the surest foundation for raising children and remains the choice of the majority of people in Britain. We want to strengthen the institution of marriage to help more marriages to succeed
>
> (Home Office/Ministerial Group on the Family 1998, p. 4)

and

> This government believes that marriage provides a strong foundation for stable relationships
>
> (Home Office/Ministerial Group on the Family 1998, p. 30)

The government advocates a 'third way' that offers a compromise between those for whom marriage is the bedrock of 'the family' and those for whom it has become just one among many forms of family life.

CONCLUSION

Family policy is difficult to define and subject to heated debate. Whether family policy is broadly or narrowly conceived, and oriented to implicit or explicit aims, it is likely to prove controversial because of the issues it raises. These we discussed in terms of the basic family activities which form the framework of this book: reproduction, socialization, care and protection, distribution and work. Controversies arise in large measure from the problems of adapting family policies to rapid changes in experiences and expectations in all of these activities. The debate over family values in the mid-1990s reflected growing uncertainties about what roles the family should play, and how its responsibilities should be regulated.

To clarify this debate, we classified perspectives on family policy in terms of ends (traditional, egalitarian and pragmatist) and means (interventionist and libertarian). Combining these classifications produces a framework within which we can try to identify family policies. For example, if we take New Labour at face value, we might classify it as interventionist and pragmatist.

	Traditional	Egalitarian	Pragmatist
Interventionist			New Labour?
Libertarian			

However, while classification can indicate the fault lines along which perspectives divide, it tends to exaggerate the degree of uniformity in policy positions. Contradictory policies are often pursued within the same political perspective. The Conservative governments of the 1980s and 1990s supported home ownership, while obliging people to sell off the 'family home' to pay for long-term care. It stressed the importance of making young people 'independent' while forcing them to rely increasingly upon family support. Such contradictions reflect the realities of policy-making, which is often less a rational and comprehensive appraisal of alternatives than an incremental response to immediate problems and pressures or an exploitation of opportunities for short-term political advantage.

KEY POINTS

- Defining 'family' varies by cultural values, relationships, countries, times and purposes.
- There is no agreed definition of family policy; it may be implicit or explicit in its aims, comprehensive or selective in scope, and coherent or unco-ordinated across different policy areas.
- Approaches to family policy differ in their ends, which can be traditionalist, egalitarian or pragmatist; their means and values, which can be libertarian or interventionist; their institutional form and how they fit into the structures of government; and in how they see the relationship between the family and state.
- Family policy includes policies to distribute or redistribute resources within or between families; policies to regulate behaviour of family members; and policies to create or modify the procedures and structures through which distribution and regulation operate.
- Family policy is linked to wider social policy discourses and agendas, distinguished by whether policies are oriented to meeting the needs of families, managing or resolving family problems, or recognizing the rights of family members.

GUIDE TO FURTHER READING

For a very good brief introduction to family policy, see:

Millar, J. (1998) 'Social policy and family policy' in Alcock, P., Erskine, A. and May, M. (eds) (1998) *The Student's Companion to Social Policy*, Oxford: Blackwell and the Social Policy Association.

For the debates about key family policy and parenting issues for the 1990s, see:

Utting, D. (1995) *Family and parenthood: supporting families, preventing breakdown: a guide to the debate*, York: Joseph Rowntree Foundation.

For an examination of family change and the relationship between families and the state in Britain, see:

Harding, L. F. (1996) *Family, State and Social Policy*, Basingstoke: Macmillan.

For a comparative perspective in family policy, see:

Kamerman, S. B. and Kahn, A. J. (eds) (1997) *Family change and family policies in Great Britain, Canada, New Zealand, and the United States*, Oxford: Clarendon Press. See especially Part 1 for a review of family policy in Great Britain, by Ringen and colleagues.

Hantrais, L. and Letablier, M. (1996) *Families and Family Policies in Europe*, London: Longman.

Hantrais, L. (1995) *Social Policy in the European Union*, Basingstoke: Macmillan, Chapter 1, 'Family Policies' pp. 79–101.

Gauthier, A. H. (1996) *The State and the Family: a Comparative Analysis of Family Policies in Industrialized Countries*, Oxford: Clarendon Press.

Reproduction: trends, debates and family policies

2

Outline

Many of the concerns of family policy over reproduction focus on the issue of fitness for parenthood. In this chapter, we review concerns over cohabitation, and whether this means a decline in the stability and commitment which families can provide. Much of the debate over co-habitation is fuelled by concern over the decline of marriage, and anxiety reaches fever pitch with relation to extra-marital births, particularly to teenage mothers. This is not conducive to a cool appraisal of the available evidence on either cohabitation or extra-marital births. The focus on the problems associated with the decline in the traditional family tend to obscure questions of need (for example, in relation to contraception for teenagers) and of rights (notably of cohabiting couples). The issue of rights is especially vexed in relation to adoption, where the rights of children, adoptive parents and natural parents may be hard to reconcile. New reproductive technologies have posed a further set of challenges to assumptions about fitness for parenting, most obviously in relation to the rights of same-sex couples to reproduce through IVF. Obsessed with concerns over marriage and the traditional family, family policy has barely begun to confront the choices arising from social and technological change.

REPRODUCTION

Reproduction is the activity we identify most closely with families, and reproductive issues tend to figure prominently in the political agenda. Family policies have been concerned with the number of babies born, where they are born, the type of families into which they are born and who conceives them.

CHANGING FERTILITY AND FAMILY STRUCTURE

Fertility patterns in Britain have been changing, with fewer children born, later child-bearing and more children born outside marriage. Similar changes have occurred in other European and North American societies.

- Women are having smaller families.
- More women are having children in their thirties.
- More women are choosing not to have children.
- More children are born outside marriage.

Family sizes have been declining for more than a century. Women are deferring having children and completed family sizes are reducing. The average family size in Britain and other European countries now stands below the level required to replace their populations. More women are remaining childless, with much of this increase due to choice.

Despite falling fertility, pro-natalist policies aimed to increase fertility and family size, common in Europe in the 1930s, have not re-emerged. This is perhaps because they have not proved very effective in influencing family size. Fertility rates have been especially low in Germany despite generous provision for mothers who stay at home to look after children. In France they remained low despite higher rates of family allowance for third and subsequent children (and no allowance for the first child). Pro-natalist policies have to compete with other factors influencing fertility. They have given way to (selective) policies for preventing rather than encouraging births, superseded by concerns over how families are formed, and who forms them.

Reproduction through marriage

Much of the contemporary debate about the family focuses on marriage, and its role in family life. Labour's *Supporting Families* (Home Office/Ministerial Group on the Family 1998) emphasizes the importance of marriage as 'the surest foundation' for family life. The Conservative Party has launched a 'crusade for the family' focused on improving tax incentives for marriage and creating obstacles to divorce. Marriage provides a means of regulating reproduction – and, more generally, of sexual activity. As only individuals above a certain age can marry, reproduction within marriage discourages early childbirth. As marriage involves two partners, parents can divide (or share) responsibilities for childcare and maintenance. As only heterosexual partners can marry, marriage regulates the sexual identities and relationships of parents.

Marriage embodies a variety of controls over reproduction to encourage it to proceed within a 'socially acceptable' framework. Traditionally it provided a method of enforcing responsibility on fathers – hence the 'shotgun' wedding in an age when mothers had little control over pregnancy and childbirth. The responsibility imposed on fathers to become breadwinners was matched by an obligation on mothers to become home-makers. In the nineteenth century, those mothers not conforming to this stereotype were expected to support themselves – although it was difficult to obtain even a subsistence wage. The state offered indoor relief (through the workhouse) or outdoor relief, but subject to various forms of social control. In affirmation of prevailing moral values, the treatment of unmarried mothers was notably harsh.

As motherhood is often treated as synonymous with marriage, marriage can provide a means of limiting and controlling female aspirations. Feminists have criticized the institution of marriage, notably the implication of distinctive reproductive roles for men and women, and the sexual division of labour in the household. Both limit women's opportunities in the public sphere and relegate them to the lower status 'private' sphere.

Marriage has even been used as a method of regulating 'race', for example through regulations on immigration (recently repealed) that required consular officials to rule on whether marriages were 'genuine' before allowing visas for entry.

However, the traditional controls that marriage exercised over reproduction have weakened. Control over contraception has given women options over the size and timing of their families, and new options in balancing the demands of home and work. They have also created opportunities for unconventional relationships and parenting by same-sex couples. Women are no longer obliged to accept a long period of child-bearing and financial dependency, and as a result the links between reproduction and marriage have weakened. Whether for good or ill has been the subject of much heated debate. We shall consider two issues which have been at the centre of these debates: cohabitation and extra-marital births.

COHABITATION

The growth of cohabitation in Britain dates at least from the early 1970s. In the mid-1960s, only 5% of couples marrying for the first time cohabited before marriage; by the 1990s 70% had cohabited (Haskey 1998, p. 23) and overall about one in eleven (9%) of those aged 16–59 were cohabiting. Clearly some period of cohabitation has become the norm for couples (Table 2.1).

Table 2.1 Percentage of women aged 18–49 cohabiting* by legal marital status: 1979–1995 Great Britain

Legal marital status**	1979 %	1995 %
Single	8	26
Separated	17	11
Divorced	20	27
Widowed	0	[8]
OVERALL	11	25

* excludes same sex cohabitees

** women described as 'separated' were legally married

[ ] estimated figure

Source: derived from ONS (1997) *Living in Britain: Preliminary results of the 1995 GHS*, London: The Stationery Office, Table A7. N = 4944.

Should policies support or discourage cohabitation? Should we remove all legal distinctions between marriage and cohabitation or between married and cohabiting parents?

Family policies have been ambivalent on these issues. Policy responses have varied in different countries, depending on the extent of cohabitation and their cultural and religious traditions. In Britain, recent policies concerning parental obligations to children adopt a neutral position on the marriage versus cohabitation debate. They are silent about marriage or cohabitation, shifting the emphasis to parental responsibilities and rights regardless of a parent's marital status. While a person might choose to avoid some of the obligations of marriage by cohabiting, a parent cannot evade their obligations towards their children simply by choosing not to marry the other parent.

However, not all distinctions between married and cohabiting parents have been removed. For example, while their range of obligations are the same, unmarried fathers have yet to acquire the same range of rights as married fathers in relation to their children when relationships break down – although change here is imminent.

A further area where family policies do not treat cohabitation in a consistent fashion can be found in tax and benefit policies. The British social security system usually treats cohabiting couples as a family unit where this restricts entitlement to benefit, and denies recognition where this would establish rights to benefit to which married couples do not have access. The 1966 Social Security Act required the resources of cohabiting couples, those living as husband and wife, to be aggregated when assessing benefit entitlement, whether or not such aggregation actually takes place. Whether cohabitation constitutes 'living as husband and wife' is ascertained through the application of a number of guidelines. These include such factors as co-residence, the stability of the relationship, mutual financial support, sexual relations, the care of children, and public recognition – although none of these in isolation may establish that a couple are living together 'as husband and wife'. However, cohabitees do not have all the benefits available to married couples, such as the rights to survivor's social security benefits. This approach is one which continues to privilege marriage, while recognizing the fact of cohabitation in some respects.

It has been argued that some features of the tax and benefit system favoured cohabitees, and acted as a disincentive to marriage. These features have been gradually modified so as to remove any financial advantage cohabitation might have held over marriage. For example, the larger mortgage interest tax relief on loans for owner-occupied housing that had been available to cohabitees has now been removed. On the other hand, all the opportunities for tax efficiencies available to married couples have not been fully extended to cohabitees.

Finally, it is not only in public policy but also in family law that partial recognition of cohabitation can be found. For example, cohabitees have been given some but not all of the remedies for domestic violence and occupancy rights in the family home that are available to married spouses. However, recognition of cohabitation has been much more limited with regard to rights to inherit from a partner, rights to remain in a family home, or rights to the property (or pension) of a partner when a relationship breaks down.

Trends in cohabitation

The debate about cohabitation has been driven by different interpretations of cohabitation as a social trend. Is it a threat to marriage, a complement to marriage or a viable alternative to marriage? What does the evidence tell us?

In Britain, cohabitation still seems more a prelude to marriage than a replacement of it. High rates of cohabitation among those in their late twenties and early thirties reflect a delay in marriage rather than a decline in its appeal. The trend to later first marriage (Table 2.2) is due in some part to time spent cohabiting beforehand.

Table 2.2 Mean age of first marriage 1961–1998

	Men	Women
1961	25.6	23.1
1981	25.4	23.1
1991	27.5	25.5
1996	29.7	27.7
1998*	30.0	27.7

* estimate

Source: ONS 1999, p.93

Cohabitation can also be seen as a prelude to re-marriage, most obviously when re-marriage must be delayed until one of the partners is divorced. Very similar proportions of single (26%) and divorced (27%) women were cohabiting in 1995 (ONS 1997: Table A7).

This interpretation of cohabitation is supported by evidence on its durability (Table 2.3).

Table 2.3 The duration of cohabitation 1989 Great Britain

	Women		
	Single	Separated/divorced	All cohabitants
1 year or less	32	31	32
2 years or less but more than 1 year	23	20	22
5 years or less but more than 2 years	32	28	29
Over 5 years	13	21	22
Median duration in months	21	24	22

Source: 1989 GHS data, quoted in Kiernan and Estaugh (1993) Table 2.5

Most cohabiting relationships are relatively short-lived, because the couple either split up or get married. The great majority of cohabitations either end or progress to marriage within 5 years; only 16% of female cohabitees had cohabited for more than 5 years.

Perhaps the chief significance of cohabitation, then, is as a stage in partnership and family formation, replacing a period of formal engagement. However, alternative interpretations of the evidence are possible. Traditionalists might interpret the short duration of cohabiting partnerships as an indicator of their intrinsic instability. Married couples who cohabit are more likely to separate or divorce within 15 years than those who have not. Those who cohabit with one partner prior to marriage form unions no less stable than those who marry before living together. But serial cohabitation (cohabiting with a series of partners) prior to marriage is associated with marital instability. While this may simply reflect disenchantment with conventional relationships, it has been taken as evidence of irresponsibility in personal relationships and a reluctance to fulfil essential roles and responsibilities, notably to children.

The growth in cohabitation may reflect a decline in the supply of males capable of playing the role of family 'breadwinner'. Improving economic fortunes may weaken or even reverse the trend towards cohabitation. Cohabitation is one solution to problems posed by long-term labour market change, which has reduced the pool of eligible men and increased the prospects of self-sufficiency for women. Evidence suggests that cohabitation is related more to declining male fortunes than any improvement in female prospects. A large majority of long-term cohabitees live in disadvantaged socio-economic circumstances: poorly educated, often unemployed, living in state housing and dependent on state benefits, with few assets to bequeath. The growth in cohabitation among the single (never married) slowed significantly during the early to mid-1990s, while rates among the separated and divorced actually declined (ONS 1997). Nevertheless the Office for National Statistics estimates that the number of people co-habiting in England and Wales may double over the next 25 years (from 1.56 million in 1996) with the most dramatic rise among older couples.

Cohabitation and childbirth

Is the growth in cohabitation evidence of an increasing separation of marriage and childbearing? Most cohabitation is childless, although about one in three cohabitees live in households with dependent children (perhaps of previous relationships), and the trend is for more children to be born to a cohabiting couple and grow up with parents not legally married to each other.

A qualitative study by McRae (1993) tried to assess the link between cohabitation and motherhood. McRae interviewed 328 mothers who had been or were cohabiting. McRae asked these mothers why they cohabited, and why they married or continued to cohabit. She found little to differentiate cohabiting mothers who married before giving birth from those who did not. Even among long-term cohabitees, women tended to marry for similar reasons, and when they married reflected pragmatic considerations, such as whether they could afford it, or were waiting for a divorce. The family lives of cohabitees were similar to those of married couples. Cohabiting partners tended to be more egalitarian in outlook and attitudes. But when it came to the practicalities of sharing tasks, or happiness with their relationships, views and experiences were very similar. There was little to choose between them when it came to fulfilling responsibilities – even when partnerships broke down. Having children tended to have a greater impact on family life than whether or not the partners were legally tied. Overall, McRae found little evidence to suggest that cohabitation was undermining marriage – even among those who became mothers while cohabiting.

BIRTHS OUTSIDE MARRIAGE

Traditionalists are even more alarmed at the rise in children being born outside marriage and in children growing up in households headed by cohabiting partners or a single, never married, mother. The proportion of births outside marriage maintained a fairly steady level of about 5% to 7% of all births until the 1960s. Extra-marital childbearing rose sharply between 1976 and 1995, from 9% to 34%.

Although the numbers of all lone-parent families has grown sharply since 1971, the most rapidly growing group has been single mothers – those never legally married (Table 2.4). Divorce and separation remain the main routes into lone parenthood (for a majority of lone parents), but by 1992, single mothers accounted for 35% of lone-parent families – almost half a million single mothers caring for over 1.5 million children.

Table 2.4 Family type and marital status of lone mothers: 1971–1996
Families with dependent children+ Great Britain

Family type	1971		1996	
	%		%	
Married couple++	92		79	
Lone mother	7		20	
single		1		7
widowed		2		1
divorced		2		6
separated		2		5
Lone father	1		2	
All lone parents	8		21	

+ dependent children are persons under 16, or aged 16–18 and in full-time education, in the family unit, and living in the household
++ including married women whose husbands were not defined as resident in the household

Source: ONS (1998)

The latest figures show that in England and Wales half of all conceptions in 1997 took place outside marriage (400,000 of 800,000 conceptions). Fewer extra-marital conceptions result in births, but even so a growing proportion of births are outside marriage; increasing from 8% in 1971 to 13% in 1981 to 34% in 1995. An increasing number of births are to mothers who have never married.

The rate of teenage pregnancy in the UK is the highest in western Europe, although the latest figures suggest that the rate may be falling, down 1% between 1996 and 1997 with under-age pregnancies falling 5% in the same period.

With reference to Table 2.5, we can see how teenage motherhood has changed.

Table 2.5 Live births to women under the age of 20 1951–1992

Year	Total births (000s)	Rate (1)	Births outside marriage (000s)	Rate (2)	% of live births outside marriage
1951	29.1	21	4.8	3.7	16
1961	59.8	37	11.9	8.0	20
1971	82.6	51	21.6	14.6	26
1981	56.6	28	26.4	13.2	41
1991	52.4	33	43.4	28.0	83
1992	47.9	32	40.1	–	84

Source: adapted from Selman and Glendinning (1996, p. 204), quoting OPCS Birth Statistics

Rate (1) is per 1,000 women aged 15–19
Rate (2) is per 1,000 single, divorced or widowed women 15–19

However, most births are co-registered by the child's mother and father, the majority of whom give the same address (Table 2.6). Of births outside marriage in 1995, 60% were jointly registered by parents living at the same address at the time of the birth, and another fifth by both parents living at different addresses. The proportion of births registered only by the mother has hardly grown at all. Jointly registered births account for about 90% of the increase in extramarital births.

Table 2.6 Teenage births outside marriage, by registration 1964–1991

Year	Total births	Sole registration (%)	Joint registration (%)
1964	17.4	81	19
1971	21.6	72	28
1981	26.4	52	48*
1991	43.4	35	65*

Source: adapted from Selman and Glendinning (1996, p. 205), quoting OPCS Birth Statistics

*The majority of joint registrations were from the same address.

Thus a common route into single motherhood is now likely to be because of a cohabitation that has broken down. Thus, 'single' parents may be 'single' only in a legal, but not a de facto, sense. One estimate suggests that more than 40% of single mothers may have been in cohabiting partnerships that broke down. It cannot be inferred that 'single' parenthood involves the complete absence of fathers. Single mothers are a heterogeneous group who do not conform in general to the popular image of young mothers choosing to have children on their own, without the involvement of fathers.

The political response

Nevertheless, the growth of single motherhood provoked a storm of controversy. In 1993 Conservative ministers attacked the social irresponsibility of unmarried mothers, suggesting that they should be denied welfare benefits and access to council housing, and advocating a return to adoption as 'the best outcome'. Although somewhat less hysterical, New Labour too sees the growth of lone parenthood as a social problem, notably in regard to social exclusion and the high costs of welfare dependency. The Labour government has also made headlines of the 'Ministers to take harsh line on single mothers' and 'Mothers urged to give up babies' variety (Grice 1999 and Jury and Burrell 1999, both in *The Independent*).

Why has the political establishment (both Conservative and Labour) become so alarmed? One explanation may lie in a misleading interpretation of the statistics. If no distinction is drawn between teenage mothers, single mothers and lone parents, the scale of the 'problem' is readily exaggerated. In fact, although four in five teenage mothers are single parents they constitute only 4% of all lone mothers. And they may not be single for long. Half the teenage mothers in a recent NCDS study went on to live with the father of their child (Kiernan 1995). Although its duration is increasing, single parenthood is usually a temporary state which lasts on average for a shorter period (about 3 years) than other forms of lone parenthood (about 5 years).

One concern shared by the political establishment centres on the economic viability of single-parent families. Single parents tend to have a low income – even relative to that of lone mothers as a whole. In 1994 more than half (57%) had a gross household income of less than £100 a week. By contrast, 62% of married couples enjoyed gross household incomes in excess of £350 a week (OPCS 1996 Table 2.20).

These low incomes reflect low rates of participation in paid employment among single mothers. Of single mothers, 57% were not in paid employment in 1994 compared with 50% of all lone mothers and 31% of married mothers (OPCS 1996 Table 2.18). Of single mothers whose youngest child was under 5, only 11% had part-time jobs in 1992–1994, compared with 15% of all lone mothers and 36% of married mothers (OPCS 1996 Table 2.19). Single mothers are especially dependent on benefit, with 90% of young single mothers (and 82% of those over 25) relying on Income Support. Here then lies the rub. With the social security budget under pressure, the rise in the population of single mothers reliant on Income Support is seen as a major problem.

The social characteristics of young mothers also render them vulnerable, both socially and politically. Kiernan (1995) using NCDS data found low educational attainment was the most powerful factor associated with becoming a young parent. Early parenthood was more common where school performance was static or declined over time. Young parents were more likely to come from families with low socio-economic status in financial difficulties. The chances of becoming a teenage mother were higher for those whose own mother gave birth as a teenager, and for those who experienced emotional difficulties during childhood and adolescence. This evidence suggests that single parenthood is associated with economic and social vulnerability, especially among the young.

The 'problem' of single parenthood

While so much is common ground, there are divisions over the explanations and implications of the rise in single parenthood. Those preaching traditional 'family values' tend to see single parenthood mainly as a moral problem rooted in self-interest and irresponsibility. Young mothers are accused of using extra-marital births to secure housing or benefits. Young fathers are accused of failing to accept parental (and especially financial) responsibility for their off-spring. Children brought into the world and brought up (or neglected) by 'irresponsible' parents, it is argued, are themselves less likely to conform to traditional values or achieve respectability in terms of education and employment. The absence of fathers is seen as undermining the proper socialization of children, particularly boys, into acceptable forms of social behaviour.

Several arguments have been made in defence of single parents. One concerns the need to look at how families evolve across time, particularly in relation to the role of fathers. Some of the other assumptions about the motivations and attitudes of teenage mothers have been challenged by qualitative evidence.

One in-depth study found little evidence to support the contention that teenage mothers use pregnancy as a means of securing housing or benefits (Phoenix 1991). A survey of lone parents in 1993 found only 1% of all single lone parents had planned their child and given some weight to housing prospects in doing so – and half of these had a long wait after birth before being housed (Ford *et al.* 1995, p. 88). In another study, Speak *et al.* (1995) found that women coming forward as homeless or threatened with homelessness were genuinely in great distress.

There is evidence that young mothers conceive not because of ignorance or design – but as a result of complex and contradictory feelings associated with the use of contraception (Phoenix 1991). Another qualitative study of 31 unmarried mothers who were teenagers at conception suggests that young single motherhood was not planned. Conceptions occurred despite contraception as well as without it, and women chose not to have abortions partly out of moral conviction (Burghes and Brown 1995). Other evidence could find no girls aged 16–17, and only 4% of those aged 18–19, who rejected contraception because of dislike, habit or a desire to become pregnant (Office for National Statistics 1997 Table 11.5).

On the other hand, the qualitative evidence does suggest that young mothers have serious difficulties in setting up home, both in relation to housing and income. It reveals the importance of family support for young mothers, both emotional and practical – but also the limitations of that support, given low family incomes and the stigma still attached to extra-marital birth. Young mothers often end up with poorly furnished accommodation in poor neighbourhoods, struggling to survive on low incomes and vulnerable to any small-scale fluctuations in their requirements, such as winter clothing.

The evidence we have considered is far from conclusive – one must be cautious, for example, in extrapolating from small-scale qualitative studies conducted in particular locales. The implications are, in any case, ambiguous. The evidence does not support the more dogmatic assumptions of those for whom any departure from marriage is symptomatic of moral dereliction. Both single parents and cohabitees tend to share the aspirations and accept the responsibilities generally associated with parenthood.

Early child-bearing and cohabitation tend to be associated with low income and other resources, with attendant problems in achieving an adequate standard of living. This poses a dilemma for a society which is increasingly disposed (at least in rhetoric) to recognize the interests and rights of children. A more punitive approach to cohabitation and single parenthood, intended to provide incentives to work or marry, may be achieved at the expense of the children while having little effect on deep-rooted social trends.

Social policies and single parents

Do social policies influence the rate of young single parenthood, either positively or negatively? Selman and Glendinning (1996) review a range of social policies using comparative European and American evidence. They conclude that British welfare and housing policies do not appear to encourage teenage pregnancy, nor do they give advantageous treatment to young single mothers over other young people without children. If anything, they would have a disincentive effect on teenage motherhood since benefit levels for 16- and 17-year-old parents are lower than for those aged 18 or more, and teenage parents under 16 have no independent benefit entitlement at all. Recent changes add further disincentives to a life on benefit. Selman and Glendinning (1996) also cite research finding no evidence for the claim that young women have children in order to get housing. Comparing the levels of teenage births with levels of welfare benefits in other countries, they do not find there is a link between high rates of teenage births and generous benefits. Rather, in countries with low rates of teenage births, there appears to be more generous benefits for all families or greater encouragement for all mothers to be economically active, and teenage mothers are treated similarly to older mothers.

Nevertheless, the 1993 moral panic about unmarried teenage mothers prepared the political ground for the restriction of housing entitlement and the subsequent freezing of lone-parent benefit and the lone-parent premium paid to those on Income Support. The policy rhetoric shifted from protecting the vulnerable to penalizing the irresponsible. A more pragmatic approach might focus on the kind of factors which seem to be associated with early pregnancy, which the Social Exclusion Unit established by the Blair government identified as follows:

- young people who have been looked after by local authorities
- children whose mothers gave birth as teenagers
- some ethnic groups
- young people who are homeless
- young offenders
- those with special educational needs
- young people growing up in poverty
- poor educational attainment/attendance
- family breakdown
- informal and unreliable sex education.

Young people leaving care are disproportionately represented among teenage pregnancy figures, with over one in seven and approaching one in four young women leaving care already pregnant or already mothers, suggesting that the state might first put its own house in order. But some factors may be more amenable to intervention than others. For example, evidence suggests that the practically simple (if morally contestable) step of making a morning-after pill more freely available can have a dramatic impact on unwanted pregnancies, reducing them by one-third among a group of Edinburgh women compared with those who needed prescriptions. The 1990s have seen an 18% reduction in teenage pregnancy among under-16s, and a 13% drop in pregnancies among 15–19 year olds – which Alison

Hadley (of the Brook Advisory Clinic) attributes to the 'unprecedented expansion of services' since 1991.

Selman and Glendinning (1996) found a positive relationship between low rates of teenage births and explicit sex education policies and easy access to contraception and abortion. In countries with low teenage birth rates (the Netherlands, Sweden and Denmark), policies do not seek to restrict teenage sexual activity (which seems to be similar across all countries) but to reduce the likelihood that this will result in an unwanted pregnancy or an unplanned birth. In this respect, Childline has reported a very high level of calls from under-age girls to its helpline about pregnancy and under-age sex – suggesting a gap in agency support and practical knowledge of contraception (Murphy 1999).

However, calls for action to reduce teenage pregnancies through better advice/support are still controversial. A proposal to establish drop-in centres for information about contraception and allow nurses to prescribe contraceptive pills in schools was castigated by anti-abortion campaigners as turning nurses into 'agents of the sex industry'. The churches remain hostile to any policies that might be seen as encouraging teenagers not to abstain from sex.

The Social Exclusion Unit set up by the Labour government has made a series of proposals to tackle teenage pregnancies. These include:

- The provision of supervised hostels for young mothers (instead of local authority housing) to provide advice on parenting and support with childcare, education and employment.
- An overhaul of sex education at school, with primary schools required to have a policy on sex and relationships education, and secondary schools to provide more comprehensive sex education focusing on boys as well as girls.
- An increase in the number of school nurses, and an expansion in the role in advising how to obtain contraception.
- The pursuit of young men through the Child Support Agency to meet financial obligations regardless of age.
- A system of 'peer mentoring' with teenage mothers visiting schools to report how hard their role is.

These policies accept the educative role of information in dispelling ignorance rather than inciting sexual activity. They also emphasize the importance of moral responsibility, notably in the determination to impose financial obligations upon young fathers. On the other hand, Labour has been cautious in extending practical support by way of contraception. Although school nurses have an advisory role, the Blair government has rejected any move to allow them to prescribe contraceptives. Similarly, the Scottish government has created task forces to tackle teenage pregnancies but morning-after pills will not be made more freely available. It is also far from clear whether the proposed 'hostels' for young mothers will play a supportive rather than a traditionally punitive role.

The question of how to provide adequate social support to single parents while minimizing financial costs to the Exchequer has still to be addressed. Whether governments can reconcile an inclination to penalize irresponsibility with an adequate programme of prevention and protection for young mothers remains to be seen.

ADOPTION

Those opposed to efforts to prevent teenage pregnancies through sex education and contraception tend to look favourably on adoption as an appropriate response to single motherhood. For example, Conservative politician John Redwood in 1996 urged teenage single mothers to give their babies up for adoption. The Labour government has since urged young mothers who cannot cope with their babies to give them up for adoption. There was also Conservative talk (again taken up by the Labour government) of reintroducing hostels for single mothers – a traditional sanction presented as an educational measure to improve their fitness for parenting.

Adoption (and fostering) policies reveal assumptions about who can be considered capable parents. For example, in 1998 the government decided that adults who believe in physical punishment should be banned from fostering. Adoption policies also reflect tensions between the interests of children, natural parents, and would-be adopters. This may be why adoption has had such a high political profile despite its small scale in recent years.

Due to social changes such as the falling birthrate, wider availability of contraception and abortion, changing sexual morality and reduced stigma attached to raising children born outside marriage, the profile of adoption has changed. The number of adoptions has declined steadily and only a very small number of adoptions now involve infants biologically unrelated to either of their adoptive parents. About 25,000 children were adopted in the peak year of 1968, but by 1996 adoptions had fallen to about 6,000, including only 253 babies less than 1 year old. In Scotland, the number of adoptions recorded by the Registrar General during 1997 was 471; about half of the children were adopted by a biological parent and stepparent, and many were older children (over one-third were aged 4 or older) or children with special needs (Edwards and Griffiths 1997, p. 167).

The legal and policy responses to these changes have involved a more open approach to adoption. There is now greater recognition that adopted children should receive support in continuing attachments with their birth families, when feasible, and that there should be greater openness in tracing birth families. Adoption is increasingly seen primarily as a means to meet the needs of children, rather than as simultaneously meeting the needs of childless couples. Open policies such as these challenge traditional conceptions of family boundaries. However, tensions remain over the use of adoption, given the potentially conflicting interests of biological parents and prospective adoptees, and children may be unhappily caught in the middle, in the form of local authority care.

Mixed-race adoption

The tensions over adoption are given a 'racial' twist when the children of ethnic minority mothers are considered for adoption by 'white' adoptive parents. For 'black' professionals in particular, this could seem tantamount to the removal of children from ethnic minority parents suffering discrimination and disadvantage, to satisfy the desires of childless but otherwise advantaged 'whites' couples. Many local authorities (Lambeth Council led the field) introduced or practised 'same-race' adoption policies, on the grounds that the racial and cultural identities of 'black' children should be taken into account in selecting adoptive parents. Under the Children Act 1989, adoption was to be decided on the basis of the child's best interests, although these interests may be difficult to determine when the child and the prospective parents are of different 'ethnic' backgrounds. Since 1989 professionals in England and Wales have been obliged to take account of ethnic identity (and religion and creed), and in particular whether prospective parents show sufficient sensitivity to 'racial issues'. But this can be a difficult judgement to make.

Where prospective parents have been rejected because of 'lack of understanding of racial issues' they may see themselves as victims of 'political correctness' on the part of professionals – a perception encouraged by politicians making political capital at their expense. John Major complained that 'I still hear too many stories of politically correct absurdities that prevent children being adopted by loving couples that would give them a good home'. After some controversial cases, new regulations from April 1997 gave prospective parents rights to be better informed about the processing of their application, and to challenge a recommendation by the adoption panel. The then Health Secretary, Stephen Dorrell, suggested that:

> Decisions about which parents are able to adopt children should reflect common-sense values that are widely shared throughout society, and shouldn't reflect the rather specialist and fashionable theories of a particular professional group
>
> (cited in Cooper 1997)

However, it is by no means clear how taking account of widely shared 'common-sense' values will help determine the best interests of the child. Indeed, an appeal to common-sense values may invite stereotyped responses, based not on an individual's merits (or drawbacks) as a potential parent but on their membership of a particular group. People belong to many varied and competing groups, so it becomes a matter of identifying them through some particular characteristic (e.g. race, creed, sexual orientation) which is seen to (dis)qualify them from parenthood. For example, 'gays' may be seen as 'sensitive' and 'caring' – or 'potentially abusive'. The media seem inclined to the latter view, to judge by the fuss attending the fostering of an 11-year-old boy by a gay couple. But Anya Palmer (spokeswoman for Stonewall) argues that 'it's not a good idea to make judgements about people as members of a group rather than as individuals'.

Labour's policies

Disputes over adoption illustrate the variety of pressures which can influence family policy. Politicians and the professionals have frequently clashed over the use of adoption, reflecting different views over the fitness of potential parents. Albeit in more muted tones, the Labour government is also planning to challenge an 'anti-adoption culture' of professional social work, to which it attributes the very wide variation in adoption levels among different local authorities, and the large numbers of children who remain in public care for long periods.

The Labour government has focused on relatively low rates of adoption among some local authorities. Only 2,000 of 50,000 children in care are adopted each year. The government is introducing new targets to ensure fewer children remain in local authority care for long periods, and it aimed to spend £30 million in 1999 to develop better procedures and choice of placement, including closer inspection and regulation of standards of care and adoption services.

These measures are intended to shift the emphasis from institutional care towards adoption. They are approved by those like Julian Brazier, the Conservative MP for Canterbury and founder of a pro-adoption group of MPs, who believe there is an 'anti-adoption culture' in some local authorities. A House of Commons survey showed that adoption rates are very low among some authorities, particularly Labour-led London boroughs, with Ealing for example placing in adoption only one of the 393 children in its care during 1997. On the other hand, those involved in adoption procedures might explain low adoption rates in terms of high numbers of difficult-to-place children and the need – since adoption is for life – to ensure an 'exact' match between child and family.

NEW REPRODUCTIVE TECHNOLOGIES

At the same time as family forms have diversified, so too have the means by which one can become (or avoid becoming) a parent. Technological advances have produced a succession of new reproductive options. These have widened the potential pool of individuals who may become parents, and also the dilemmas facing potential parents. The question of 'Who is fit to become a parent?' is asked with ever greater anxiety, regarding an ever diversifying population of prospective parents.

It is easier to pose the question, however, than to identify whether or how it should be answered – and by whom. Politicians and the media have not been slow to volunteer their opinions, but assumptions about the 'fitness' of parents are also implicit in welfare administration – in the rules which govern benefit entitlement, the care interventions of local authority social workers over child protection, or judgements by medical practitioners and health boards about access to 'in vitro' treatment. Thus the state has a stake in judging the fitness of parents, or rather, the state has several stakes, if we recall the diverse interests and ideologies of the politicians, professionals, and bureaucrats whose activities compose this complex and ever-changing entity.

As technology opens up new avenues to conception and parenthood, it poses challenges to cultural assumptions about supposedly 'natural' methods of conception. Should fertility treatments be provided free on the NHS – and to whom should they be made available? Should insemination be allowed after the death of a partner, as successfully claimed by Diane Blood following the death of her husband? Should donor insemination involving 'mixed race' genes be allowed? Should donor insemination be available to single women or lesbian couples? Should medically-assisted conceptions be made available to older women? Should parents be allowed to choose the sex of a child? Who is the legal parent? Do egg or sperm donors or surrogate mothers have any parental obligations? Are commercial surrogacy arrangements or other forms of financial compensation acceptable? Do we owe an obligation of care to future children to decide on the fitness of their prospective parents? What rights do children have to know their biological origins? And if the technology becomes available, should adults be allowed to reproduce themselves through clones?

Technology can limit as well as liberate, if those who seek to benefit from its power can neither afford nor control it. The means to enable conception have not become as freely available as the means to prevent it. The price of in vitro fertilization (IVF) treatment can be substantial; up to £10,000 – the cost of treatment offered by one British doctor (to enable parents to select the sex of their child). With an average success rate of 14%, repeat treatments may be necessary and even then, success may not be assured. If society is expected to meet some of this cost, then this inevitably increases the stake which 'society' has in issues of reproduction, and provides a legitimation for the state to intervene in such matters. Whether society is prepared to meet these costs depends partly on how far reproduction is defined as a 'need'. For example, in the case of IVF, a need has to be established not only to treat infertility but also to allow women (or couples) to have 'a child of their own' – meaning a child genetically linked to its parent(s). Such needs may seem 'natural' but may be culturally formed. Van Dyck (1995, pp. 61–85) for example argues that the 'need' for IVF was constructed largely through medical and media discourses focusing on a largely mythical 'infertility epidemic', allied to the 'naturalization' of IVF as a fertility treatment. Thus apparently 'natural' needs may be identified and defined within given cultural and political contexts.

A policy response to these developments and dilemmas was inevitable. The Warnock Report (1984) set out the broad foundation for the subsequent legislation, the Human Fertilisation and Embryology Act 1990. It established a regulatory framework and an executive agency, the Human Embryology and Fertilisation Authority (HEFA). That framework includes the licensing of clinics that may offer fertility treatment, and the requirement that access to assisted parenthood must take account of the welfare of any child subsequently born, including its need for a father. Other factors that can be considered include any potential risks to a child, and parental motivations, health and age. In the case of insemination following the death of the donor (which requires their prior written consent in Britain) questions are raised about whether the rights and desires of adults (to have a child by the deceased) are taking precedence over the rights and welfare of the child. Such considerations have led to a series of headline cases – 'Concern over babies born to fathers beyond the grave' is a typical example (Norton 1999) – where treatment has been questioned or denied due to age, disability, or sexual orientation. While age limits may have some medical justification, it is clear that social considerations also influence decisions about treatment.

CONCLUSION

In the midst of such uncertainties, we can at least be sure that changing family structures will increasingly diversify the family settings in which reproduction occurs, and will continue to present new issues and challenges for family policies. This chapter has underlined the difficulties which societies and governments experience in adjusting to rapid change. As we have seen in the case of cohabitation, these difficulties stem in part from the problem of interpreting trends. Problems of interpretation are compounded by the clash of rival perspectives, with cohabitation alternatively praised (if libertarian) or pilloried (if traditionalist) without much regard to evidence. This is even more evident in the case of extra-marital births, where it has often proved easier to score political points than to produce practical policies. The twists and turns which have marked the evolution of adoption policies also reflect the difficulties of identifying, let alone reconciling, the competing interests at stake. In the application of new reproductive technologies (NRT), a further set of challenges has emerged to prevailing conceptions of who is fit to reproduce. In all these cases – cohabitation, extra-marital births, adoption and NRT – the sheer pace and force of social change forces us to consider whether and how to maintain or adjust traditional conceptions of appropriate reproductive roles.

KEY POINTS

- Changing British family structures create challenges for family policy. The most important changes are:
  - fewer children are being born and family sizes are smaller
  - fewer people are marrying
  - more children now grow up, for part of their childhood, in lone-parent families or stepfamilies
  - more cohabitation before or between marriages
  - child-bearing is later
  - more women remain voluntarily childless
  - more extra-marital births
  - the association between parenthood and marriage is weaker.
- Family policies related to reproduction focus on the type of families into which children are born, the stability or otherwise of non-traditional families, and the support they should get.
- Family policies are ambivalent about the role of marriage in family life and whether its alternatives represent a threat to children and society.
- Despite its small scale recently, adoption is controversial since policies imply assumptions about fitness for parenting and family boundaries. Adoption policies now focus on children's needs and are more open about birth families.

- New reproductive technologies have diversified the ways of becoming a parent. Access to these is informed by assumptions about fitness for parenting.

GUIDE TO FURTHER READING

For discussions of changing family demography, see:

David, M. E. (ed.) (1998) *The Fragmenting Family: does it matter?*, London: IEA (Institute for Economic Affairs Health and Welfare Unit). Changing family demography is traced by Haskey, with commentaries from traditional and pragmatic perspectives (Morgan and Kiernan).

Kamerman, S. B. and Kahn, A. J. (eds) (1997) *Family change and family policies in Great Britain, Canada, New Zealand, and the United States*, Oxford: Clarendon Press, pp. 34–46.

For a traditionalist perspective on family policy, see:

Morgan, P. (1995) *Farewell to the Family? Public Policy and Family Breakdown in Britain and the USA*, London: IEA.

For a pragmatic perspective on family policy, see:

Coote, A., Harman, H. and Hewitt, P. (1998) 'Family Policy: Guidelines and Goals' in Franklin, J. (ed.) (1998) *Social Policy and Social Justice*, Cambridge: Polity Press (with IPPR), extracts from the 1990 IPPR publication, *The Family Way*.

For a discussion of adoption, see:

Ryburn, M. (1996) 'Adoption in England and Wales: current issues and future trends' in Hill, M. and Aldgate, J. (eds) (1996) *Child Welfare Services: Developments in law, policy, practice and research*, London: Jessica Kingsley, pp. 196–211.

For examinations of lone parenthood and single parenthood, see:

Bradshaw, J. (1998) 'Lone parents' in Alcock, P., Erskine, A. and May, M. (eds) (1998) *The Student's Companion to Social Policy*, Oxford: Blackwell and the Social Policy Association, pp. 263–269.

Burghes, L. (1993) *One parent Families: Policy options for the 1990s*, York: Joseph Rowntree Foundation.

Burghes, L. and Brown, M. (1995) *Single Lone Mothers: Problems, Prospects and Policies*, London: Family Policy Studies Centre.

For discussions on cohabitation, see:

McRae, S. (1993) *Cohabiting mothers: changing marriage and motherhood?* London: Policy Studies Institute.

Kiernan, K. and Estaugh, V. (1993) *Cohabitation, Extra-marital Childbearing and Social Policy,* London: Policy Studies Institute.

Socialization 3

Outline
The family continues to play a pivotal role in socialization. However, the debate over 'family values' has raised concern over its effectiveness in socializing children, and paved the way for a more interventionist approach on the part of the state. Parenting in particular has been perceived as a problem requiring remedial action, through more advice or regulation by the state. But whether the state can play an effective role in advising or regulating parents is itself open to question. The perception of young people as a 'social problem' encourages a managerial approach, most obvious perhaps in New Labour's New Deal, which imposes benefit penalties on young people refusing offers of training or work. The erosion of social rights of young people and a shift from state to family support has occurred despite evidence that they often face more difficult and fragmented transitions to adulthood. Much of the debate on socialization has instead concerned family forms, attributing deficiencies in socialization mainly to family disruption and in particular the absence of fathers. However, the search for simple 'explanations' and 'solutions' to social problems has not included close scrutiny of evidence on complex social processes involved in family transitions.

THE SOCIALIZATION OF CHILDREN

> The only function of the family that matters is socialisation
> (Lasch 1977, p. 130)

> Wherever possible, governments should offer support to all parents so that they can better support children, rather than trying to substitute for parents. There needs to be a clear understanding of the rights and responsibilities that fall to families and to governments. Parents raise children, and that is how things should remain. More direct intervention should only occur in extreme circumstances
> (Home Office/Ministerial Group on the Family 1998, p. 4)

While we associate reproduction primarily with families, the socialization of children is shared between families and other social institutions. This was not always so, but developed as economic production moved from the home to factory and office, and as educational responsibilities were assumed by school and college. Family responsibilities have shifted towards a shared or partnership role as far as the socialization of children is concerned. With the development of formal pre-school and after-school childcare, a further displacement occurs. According to Becker these displacements take place because 'many family functions in traditional societies are more effectively handled by markets and other organisations of modern societies' (cited Robertson 1991, p. 157). Others have been more critical of 'the invasion of the family by the marketplace' and the loss of 'a protected space in which to raise children' free from the 'calculating, manipulative spirit' of business life (Lasch cited Robertson 1991, p. 155). But whether one condones or condemns, clearly the family no longer serves as the sole means for the socialization of children.

Nevertheless, families continue to play a major (perhaps the major) role in socialization, and make a substantial contribution to children's education. The family remains a key learning environment for children across all social backgrounds. The strong relationship between family background and educational success has survived successive reorganizations of the educational system (Ward 1997a). It is not that schools do not make a difference (as some pessimists presume) but rather that the difference that they can make depends on how families interact with the educational process. This leaves critics divided – between those who praise the functional role of the family in the acquisition of acquiring social status and position, and those who condemn its involvement in reproducing the social divisions of class and gender. But on both sides, there is particular concern with the children who fail in – or are failed by – the process of socialization.

The 'failing' metaphor favours finding fault. Who or what can be blamed for the failures in socialization, dramatized most tragically in recent cases of murder by children? In recent years, socialization issues have revolved around questions of family form and parental responsibility. Concerns with the context for reproduction spill over into controversies about the context for subsequent socialization. For example, Charles Murray's underclass thesis locates the cause of major social ills in a failure of parents living in particular family types to socialize children adequately:

> When a large proportion of the children in a given community grows up without fathers, the next generation, especially the young males in the next generation, tend to grow up unsocialized – unready to take on the responsibilities of work and family, often criminal, often violent. The effects of absent fathers are compounded by the correlations of illegitimacy with intellectual, emotional, and financial deficits among the mothers that in turn show correlations with bad parenting practices.
>
> (Murray 1999, p. 1)

Socialization of children in families raises a plethora of issues for family policy. Is parenting in trouble? Are parents no longer fulfilling their basic responsibilities for child rearing? Do parents need training and support to do their job? What support do young people need to be good enough parents, and successfully make the transition to parenthood? Do parents satisfactorily facilitate their children's transition to adulthood? Could more be done to prevent 'dysfunctional' families and foster effective parenting? Should the state play a remedial or preventative role? Does marital disruption or family transition damage the process of socialization? How have children been affected by the increase in rates of separation and divorce? What of children growing up in households with a cohabiting couple or in stepfamilies?

To address these questions, we must consider both the contexts in which children grow up and are socialized, and what parents do, since the family provides both a setting for socialization of the next generation, and a set of activities towards that end. We first consider parenting policies directed towards parents in general. We then consider two important transitions for the socialization activities of families: the transition to parenthood for young people, and the transition for children when their parents separate and divorce.

PARENTING AND PARENTAL RESPONSIBILITY

What makes a 'good enough' parent and what contribution can family policies make to more effective parenting? These questions have been asked recently, not only by the research community but also by government policy makers. This represents a shift from a focus on problem families and poor parenting, for these questions pertain to all families. Nevertheless family policies that aim to support effective parenting still adhere to a non-interventionist stance in most cases, aiming to create a supportive framework for parenting.

Figure 3.1 Sure Start Programme, National Family and Parenting Institute and ParentLine

Faith in government support for families is evident in the Sure Start Programme, the £540 million pre-school initiative proposed in *Supporting Families* (Home Office/Ministerial Group on the Family 1998). This programme is targeted at families who, because of poor educational attainment, unemployment or other disadvantages need particular support. But some proposals are addressed to all families. As a step in providing better information, support and services for all parents, a new national agency for family research and advice, the National Family and Parenting Institute, will be set up. A free 24-hour national helpline will offer information and advice to parents. Some 250 centres for under-3s will be established to offer child-minding services, assess children at risk and provide advice on childcare. Health visitors and nursery nurses will be given an enhanced role. In essence, this will offer parents lessons in how to play with and educate their young children.

While support for effective parenting is a policy objective, there remains the problem of identifying what this is or should be. We cannot even agree on something as basic as whether children should be 'smacked' which for some is a form of physical abuse (some European countries have banned physical forms of parental punishment), and for others is reasonable chastisement and an important (and insufficiently exercised) parental responsibility. The law is increasingly involved in protecting children in what was previously viewed as a private matter. At present Scottish law recognizes parental rights to use force, but it must be moderate and not vindictive. However, UK laws are changing in favour of protecting children in response to the case of a boy caned by his stepfather, which was taken to the European Court of Human Rights.

Sex education is another important area where there is little agreement. The premise among traditionalists is that more information and more contraceptives means more young people having sex; for others, sex education means fewer unplanned pregnancies. Government guidelines state that sex education must be provided in ways which encourage young people to have regard to moral considerations and the value of family life. This moral ambivalence may mean that sex education is 'too little and too late' – researchers claim that openness about sexual matters among parents and schools is vital to young people's confidence (Moyes 1997). Comparison between British and Dutch youngsters suggests more open discussion delays the onset of sexual activity, leads to more effective use of contraception, and reduces teenage pregnancies and sexually transmitted diseases.

Figure 3.2 Good enough parents

'Good enough' parents are confident, competent parents who:

- are authoritative rather than overprotective, permissive or authoritarian
- are consistent, reliable and dependable
- offer their children love and acceptance
- set appropriate boundaries
- communicate openly and honestly
- cope with stress and deal with conflict
- avoid harsh punishment and reinforce good behaviour.

Adapted from Pugh *et al.* (1994, p. 56)

Fashions in child-rearing come and go and we cannot assume that change means 'progress'. Efforts to develop guidelines tend to present such general prescriptions that they provide a rather vague guide as to how to behave in everyday experience. For example, take the prescription that parents should be 'authoritative, rather than over protective, permissive or authoritarian' (Figure 3.2). What exactly does this mean, when it comes to deciding whether a child should be allowed out at night or if a parent should smack a child? The same issue might be raised with regard to education in parenting at schools (Figure 3.3).

Figure 3.3 Family values and guidance in schools

A National Forum for Values in Education and the Community was set up in 1996 to consider the values which ought to inform moral guidance in schools. This led to a wrangle over what to prescribe in relation to the family. The majority of the forum were content to state that families were valued 'as sources of ... support for all their members and as the basis of a society in which people care for others'. A minority statement explicitly prescribed marriage as a normative standard. A compromise was reached, and the statement of values was modified to include support for 'marriage as the traditional form of the family, whilst recognising that the love and commitment required for a secure and happy childhood can be found in families of other kinds'. The Archbishop of Canterbury later suggested that this 'can be translated into a great deal of new thinking and classroom work about the institution of marriage, why it is important, what it needs in order to flourish and what people entering marriage need to think about it'. In reply, Doug McAvoy, general secretary of the NUT, commented that teachers might lose the respect of children from lone-parent families if they 'preached that there is something wrong with their environment because they don't have two parents' (Ward 1997b).

Research on parenting suggests that this problem will not be easily resolved. Backett (1982) in her qualitative study of 22 middle class parents found that parenthood for them did not involve applying a set of rules so much as learning through trial and error. This learning process was not cumulative in that account had to be taken of the different characters and requirements of each individual child, and also reflect the different 'phases' through which children passed. Sometimes single incidents would generate a whole set of beliefs about appropriate action. What behaviour was tolerated within the family was subject to continual negotiation, with a variety of ways of coping where conflict disrupted the negotiation of acceptable behaviour. Thus parenting was an active process, rather than one determined through the application of a prescriptive set of rules to govern conduct.

In the absence of clear rules, arguments for more education of parents or regulation of parenting are open to the objection that they may impose a uniformity ill-suited to the needs of individual families. Scepticism over such 'social engineering' is fuelled by evidence of the ineffectiveness of social intervention – for example 75% of the 55,000 children in state care leave with no qualifications. Labour's introduction of late evening curfews for young children have also been criticized as an unwarranted interference with parents who should be left to get on with the job. So too might Labour's advice to parents to read to their children for 20 minutes each night – with their education spokesman, David Blunkett, reportedly advising parents 'that a story before bedtime could lead to educational success as well as being a special moment for parents and children' (Judd 1997). Yet advice to parents on 'homework' is seen as a key element in a national strategy to revolutionize literacy standards – illustrating the difficulty of drawing a sharp boundary between parental and wider social interests.

Resources for parenting

As well as raising questions concerning legitimacy and effectiveness, policy interventions to regulate parenting have been criticized for failing to address the underlying pressures which make parenting problematic. Parenting is a demanding role and good parenting needs adequate resources. Two notable issues here concern income and time. These are issues we shall return to later, so we shall confine ourselves to some brief comments here.

With regard to income, are efforts to improve parenting misconceived if they do not also address the close relationships between income inequality and social and educational disadvantage? Why focus on poor parenting given the material disadvantages of parents who are poor?

With regard to time, is effective parenting possible given the increasing constraints on 'family time' associated with longer working hours? Evidence does not suggest that participation of either or both parents in paid employment is itself a problem (Ermisch 1997). However, long hours of work are a factor influencing the extent of joint activities and participation in family life (Ferri and Smith 1996, p. 32).

Parental responsibility

Policies to 'support' effective parenting, even if presented in universal terms, can act as sticks as well as carrots, and can still target 'problem' families. The connection of poor parenting with family pathology has been reinforced by policies to hold parents responsible for socially unacceptable outcomes. The government view of parental responsibility for children's behaviour is summed up thus:

> It is neither possible nor desirable for the Government to involve itself in every aspect of family life or to dictate to parents how to raise their children: parents hold the primary responsibility for giving children the love and care they need, ensuring their welfare and security and teaching them right from wrong. But the Government can and should help parents to recognise and meet those responsibilities ...The Government is determined to reinforce the responsibility of young offenders – and their parents – for their delinquent behaviour.
>
> (Home Office 1997: para 3.2)

> Parents of young offenders may not directly be to blame for the crimes of their children, but parents have to be responsible for providing their children with proper care and control. The courts need powers to help and support parents more effectively to keep their children out of trouble
>
> (Home Office 1997: para 4.6)

Most recently, the government introduced a 'parenting order' in the Crime and Disorder Act 1998, 'designed to help and support parents in addressing their child's anti-social or offending behaviour'. Such orders (now being piloted) can be made by the courts if they consider parental attitudes and behaviour to be a key factor in child's offending. The orders can be overseen by a probation officer or a social worker, and can require parents of young offenders to enforce certain behaviours on their children or to be trained in parenting skills themselves. It is not clear what will happen if parenting orders do not produce the desired change in behaviour.

Such interventions link youth crime with 'inadequate' parenting and tend to de-emphasize the contribution of wider social factors such as poverty or unemployment. They emphasize parental control and supervision as the key parenting skills over others, and ignore the underlying constraints which may shape family life and behaviour. They also assume that models of 'good parenting' are available in terms of which promotion of good practice can proceed (O'Sullivan 1996). Thus policies tend to make assumptions about parental capacities and practice without regard to evidence – a point which applies with equal force to policies affecting the transition from childhood to adulthood.

THE TRANSITION TO ADULTHOOD

> Families are now expected to support their children throughout their teens and into their early twenties to a greater extent than ever before
>
> (Land 1996, p. 200)

Socialization begins at birth but it is less clear when it ends. The family continues to play an important socialization role into early adult life, helping young people move towards autonomy through education, into work or setting up independent homes. Family support remains important for working mothers, and teenage mothers in particular.

The growth of further and higher education (and later marriage) has tended to extend the process of children's socialization and transition to full adult status. Marriage and childbearing start later, and education finishes later. The proportion of adults completing their education at school fell from 87% in 1975 to 70% by 1995; while those completing at university rose from 2% to 9% (ONS 1997, p. 82). Young people's dependency on their families may also last longer because of their lower rates of economic activity, increased levels of unemployment, changing work patterns and declining wage rates.

Young people may remain in the parental home longer and more are returning home after a period away before finally leaving for good. The 1995 GHS survey reports a slightly reduced tendency of young single people to leave the parental home since 1979 (ONS 1997, p. 182). The National Child Development Study (NCDS) suggests that half of males and a quarter of females were living in the parental home at age 23, while 44% of men and 38% of women had returned at least once after leaving home (Jones 1995).

In the 1990s, family policies have tended to shift obligations from the state to families:

- Income Support claimants aged 18–25 receive a lower rate of benefit in the means-tested social security system.
- Minimum wages for those aged 18–21 have been set at a lower rate.
- Current funding of university education has increased the financial contribution required from many parents.

These examples illustrate the growing significance of age-related criteria in social policies, and the extent to which families, and parents in particular, are expected to provide support for an extended period while young people make the transition to work and economic independence. Dean has warned of a danger that 'eroding young people's social rights of citizenship may also corrode their sense of responsibility as citizens of the future' (Dean 1997, p. 69).

Young people are not equally able to draw on support from their families. A survey of 4,000 young Scots (Jones 1995) found only 40% of stepchildren at 18 received financial help from parents – compared with 65% of those with both biological parents at home. Jones observes that 'it is not a simple matter for young people to obtain support from their families'. Young people were sometimes suspicious of help that came with 'strings attached'; they valued their independence and preferred to avoid becoming indebted; or they did not wish to impose on their parents. The withdrawal of state support is likely, Jones argues, to increase pressures on those families who most need it.

Young people who cannot call on family support – for example, those leaving local authority care, those in conflict with parents or stepparents, those whose parents' marriages have broken down, or those whose family relationships are adversely affected by illness or violence – are especially vulnerable to homelessness and unemployment. Most of those leaving care have poor education, have no formal qualifications and are highly likely to experience unemployment. Coles (1998, p. 246) has argued that

> ... rather than receiving effective and compensatory welfare support, young people in care are subject to abuse, denied their rights and hugely disadvantaged in attempting youth transitions

The problems of young people leaving care have been given high priority by the Labour government's Social Exclusion Unit, while young people struggling to find work have been targeted by Labour's New Deal. The Labour government is reconsidering the financial support offered to 16–17 year olds, whose benefit entitlement was withdrawn by the previous government. Nevertheless it is unlikely that Labour will reverse the general trend towards greater reliance on family support, despite evidence of its limitations. Any expectation that all families will provide support is unrealistic given the prevalence of poverty and unemployment. Existing disadvantage is likely to be perpetuated and exacerbated (Morrow and Richards 1996).

Here, as in other areas of family policy, it is not at all clear where and how to draw the line between public and private responsibilities.

FAMILY 'BREAKDOWN'

Can family policy help to prevent divorce? Should family policy try to discourage divorce by making it more difficult, or to reduce conflict by removing some of the procedural barriers to divorce? The debates leading to the Family Law Act 1996 involved a clash between traditionalist, egalitarian and pragmatist perspectives over these issues. The most controversial proposals concerned extended protection from domestic violence to cohabitees and the removal of fault-based grounds for divorce such as unreasonable behaviour or adultery. Reform was driven by pragmatic concerns to reduce both the spiralling costs of civil legal aid, and conflict over divorce.

Those taking a traditionalist view found the proposal to remove 'fault' as a ground for divorce and let people divorce after 1 year's separation instead of 2 especially unpalatable. They argued that this would undermine the institution of marriage by encouraging people to take their responsibilities lightly. In their view, people ought to feel shame over divorce. To mollify such critics, Part II of the Act introduced an extended cooling-off period of 18 months; and required couples intending to divorce to attend an advisory session intended to encourage reconciliation or the use of mediation. Only once these advisory procedures were in place would 'no fault' divorce become available.

From a traditionalist perspective the state has a duty to intervene in ways which privilege marriage, while from an egalitarian view the state should intervene in ways which protect individuals regardless of marital status. From a pragmatist perspective, change in divorce law offered a means of reducing conflict on partnership breakdown (so improving the prospects for the children concerned).

It also allowed the law to be modified to take account of the growing diversity of family forms (cohabitation as well as marriage) improving the relatively vulnerable position of cohabitees.

From a pragmatist perspective, the 1996 Act could be evaluated more in terms of adjusting to and coping with the consequences of change:

> Devising policies that recognise the behavioural changes that have taken place [in families] would seem more sensible than trying to put the clock back ... Divorce is a time of acute distress for many people and parents may need considerable help and support in reaching an acceptable or best possible out come for themselves and their children.
>
> (Lewis and Maclean 1997, p. 84)

These different perspectives all share a concern with the impact of divorce on children. They all appeal to evidence of the negative outcomes of 'family breakdown' for children, but interpret that evidence in different ways.

Is the separation or divorce of parents damaging to children? Before considering the evidence that has informed policy debates, let's first set these (often heated) arguments in the context of family change, this time from the point of view of children.

The effects of family disruption on children

What kind of families do children grow up in? How have these changed over time?

Table 3.1 Children's living arrangements 1979–1991
Children aged 0–15 of women aged 18–49, Great Britain (%)

Child lives in household with:	1979	1987	1991
Both natural parents, married	83	77	68
Both natural parents, cohabiting	1	2	3
Natural mother married to stepfather	4	7	7
Natural mother cohabiting with stepfather	1	2	3
Lone mother	9	10	17
Living apart from mother	2	2	2

Source: Adapted from Clarke (1996, p. 73) from General Household Survey data

More children experience family disruption and live for at least part of their childhood in a family that does not consist of both of their married biological parents. Table 3.1 gives 'snapshots' of children's living arrangements in 3 recent years, although more children will experience life in different types of families while they are growing up. With Britain having the highest divorce rate in western Europe, in the 1980s, over one in five children (22%) experienced divorce (Clarke 1996, p. 71). The proportion of children not living with both of their married biological parents nearly doubled (from 17% to 32%) between 1979 and 1991. Older children are more likely than younger children to live in a household without one biological parent (Clarke 1996, p. 75). Children in these families can have quite complicated family networks. Nevertheless, the great majority of children live with their biological mother, and most children do still live with both of their married biological parents. Most grow up without family disruption, although it is estimated this proportion might fall to about half (Clarke 1996, p. 79).

Families today may be both more and less capable of coping with the consequences of disruption. Growing up with a lone parent, or outside a legal marriage, were equally frequent in 1851, although usually because of death rather than divorce or cohabitation. Children today have older parents, fewer siblings and a smaller kin network than in the past. This can confer benefits such as greater parental attention and material well-being, but may mean less support with childcare or when things go wrong.

Does family 'breakdown' damage children? It has been argued that marital 'breakdown' and family 'disruption' interferes with the socialization of children, adversely affecting their life chances. Even the language used – 'breakdown', 'disruption' – tends to prejudge the issue. Who would not choose an 'intact' family over one which has 'broken down'? Who would choose to be a 'lone' parent? Who would not choose a 'natural' parent? This language already presumes that some family forms are more desirable than others.

Evidence does suggest that divorce and separation produce negative outcomes for children. Survey evidence of an MRC national study of health and development in the late 1980s shows the effects of separation and divorce. Table 3.2 indicates that for children in 'manual' and 'non-manual' classes, children experiencing separation and divorce were more likely to leave school without qualifications and less likely to obtain A level or equivalent qualifications.

Table 3.2 Educational attainment of men and women by age 26 years, by social class of origin and experience of parental divorce while 0–15 years

	No qualifications %	A levels and equivalents %	Total = 100%
Males			
Manual no loss	55.0	21.0	1,049
Manual parental divorce/separation	73.0	9.5	74
Non-manual no loss	20.4	32.4	958
Non-manual parental divorce/ separation	42.4	27.3	66
Females			
Manual no loss	54.1	10.9	960
Manual parental divorce/separation	68.1	4.3	69
Non-manual no loss	19.5	34.2	888
Non-manual parental divorce/ separation	44.2	17.3	52

Source: derived from MacLean and Kuh 1991, pp. 165–166

Likewise, a study of about 1,000 young people in the west of Scotland found that children still living with both biological parents at age 15 were least likely to experience such 'negative' outcomes as use of illicit drugs, lack of qualifications, unemployment, or early pregnancy (Sweeting and West 1996). An Exeter study (Cockett and Tripp 1994) of 152 children and their parents found that children whose families had been 're-ordered' by separation or divorce were more likely than children from 'intact' families to experience lower outcomes, self-esteem, psychological health and social well-being.

Reviewing similar evidence, Utting concludes that children experiencing family breakdown 'run greater risks of educational, health and behaviour problems, compared with those whose families are intact' although adding that 'the additional risks are often modest' (Utting 1995, p. 1). Another review of research (Rodgers and Pryor 1998) also reports a range of adverse outcomes for children in separated families, including a greater chance of:

- living in poverty and in poor housing
- being poorer when adult
- behavioural problems
- needing medical treatment and experiencing depression
- poorer educational performance
- early school leaving
- early pregnancy and parenthood
- higher levels of smoking, drinking and drug use.

Nevertheless, there are problems both in interpreting this evidence, and in determining an appropriate policy response. For it is not clear what exactly produces adverse effects. Policy interventions may be more effective if they are based on sound evidence about which aspects of family disruption place children most at risk. However, it is not easy to determine what these might be.

Some evidence suggests that the form of family disruption is significant, as outcomes vary depending whether the loss of a parent is through separation or death. In the Scottish study, drug use was 20% among those with both parents, higher (37%) among those losing a parent through separation – but higher still (47%) for those losing a parent through death. Early pregnancy too was more common among those suffering separation (14%) than among those with both parents (6%) – but higher again among those losing a parent through death (40%). However, research results are inconsistent, and the impact of disruption may be mediated by other factors, such as the age of the child.

Divorce is not uniformly spread throughout the population, but is more likely to occur where educational qualifications, income level, employment history, mental health and housing are poorer. As Kiernan (1998, p. 61) observes:

> One of the challenges in assessing the legacy of divorce is being able to sort out the conditions that lead couples to separate and the potential effects on children from the consequences of the dissolution itself ... The selective nature of the population of children who experience parental divorce may lead to an overstated impression of the effects of divorce by conflating pre-existing differences amongst children from disrupted families as compared with those from non-disrupted ones, with the fall-out from marital dissolution.

Kiernan's secondary analysis (1997) of longitudinal data from a nationally representative sample of people aged 33 examined outcomes of those coming from divorce and non-divorce backgrounds. Although the divorce of parents had a negative influence, greater financial hardship and behavioural problems were evident even before the divorce took place, and these disadvantages contributed more to poorer educational attainment than the divorce itself.

Poor outcomes for children of divorced parents may be caused by factors that occur before or around the time of separation and divorce, rather than through the divorce itself. Evidence suggests that children are affected by parental conflict prior to separation and divorce. In the Sweeting and West (1996) study, those reporting more conflict with parents were more likely to have health problems and lower self-esteem. Similarly, in the Cockett and Tripp (1994) study, children in 'intact' families marked by discord between parents experienced lower outcomes for self-esteem, psychological health and social well-being than children where low levels of conflict were reported. Perhaps, then, the problem lies less in separation and divorce per se than in the parental conflicts that so often precede or attend the process of family breakdown.

We still know very little about the processes involved in how children cope with divorce and family conflict (Gano-Phillips and Fincham 1995) or the relative impact of underlying family conflict and the divorce itself on adverse outcomes for children (Rodgers and Pryor 1998). The effects of divorce may be mediated by the parental relationships sustained by divorcing partners. Robinson (1991, p. 89) identifies five types of parental relationships among divorcing couples: collaborative or collateral co-parenting, and hostile, negative or exclusive parenting by custodial parent. The quality and style of post-divorce parental relationships may have an important bearing on containing damage to children.

Arendell's study (1995) of divorced men suggests that persistent conflict between the former partners can assume priority over paternal relationships and responsibilities. Men pursuing a 'traditionalist' strategy saw themselves as 'oppressed' and marginalized by their ex-wives and in return emphasized their own rights 'at the expense of the children'. Only an innovative minority of divorced men, more secure in their identities as 'parents', were 'child-centred' and sought collaboration with ex-wives rather than resistance. Arendell argues that policies to educate men into parenting roles could have an impact in easing the conflicts precipitated by divorce. Such findings point to a positive role for initiatives to help parents to develop more constructive post-divorce relationships.

While it is clear that a good marriage is better for children than a bad divorce, but less clear whether a 'good' divorce is better for children than a 'bad' marriage. Burghes (1994, p. 48) warns that no simple relationship can be identified between marital disruption, lone parenthood and effects on children. There is no inevitable path leading from family breakdown to negative outcomes for children, since averages conceal a wide variation in individual outcomes influenced in turn by age, gender and social class. Robinson (1991, p. 89) also stresses that how divorce affects child outcomes depends on other factors, such as conflict containment and a regular positive relationship with a non-resident parent.

The emphasis in social research is gradually shifting from comparing family forms to analysing family transitions. If separation and divorce is viewed as a process rather than an event (Rodgers and Pryor 1998), it is the process of disruption and renewal and how this is handled that emerges as a key variable. Despite the value-laden language of family 'disruption' and 'renewal', this shift in perspective opens up the question of how children fare when new families are formed. We cannot assume that the loss of the previous parent is malign while the acquisition of a new (step) parent is benign. Some evidence suggests that children tend to do less well (e.g. leaving school early, or early marriage or parenthood) where children join stepfamilies (Utting 1995; Rodgers and Pryor 1998). And according to Daly and Wilson 'the presence of a step parent is the best epidemiological predictor of child abuse risk yet discovered' (cited in Morgan 1995, p. 126). While many children may benefit from steprelationships we should not automatically assume that this is so.

The options for family policy

How can these complex, incomplete and sometimes conflicting findings feed into family policies to support parents and children during family transitions? Their very complexity may make it more difficult to produce practical policy options. Moreover, it may be difficult to reconcile conflicting objectives. The findings indicate the value of minimizing parental conflict, although not how this can be done. Despite the Labour government's inclination to endorse marriage, it does emphasize the need to minimize conflict:

> When marriages run into difficulties and cannot be saved, government should ensure that the divorce process does not make the situation worse for the family as a whole by, for example, encouraging litigation or making children pawns in a fight between parents. That is why it is important to reduce conflict in divorce.
>
> (Home Office/Ministerial Group on the Family 1998, p. 37)

Various measures are proposed to further this aim, such as support for mediation on relationship breakdown, improving family support provided by court welfare services, and changing existing legal procedures to give greater clarity to the rules governing the division of family property on divorce. However, *Supporting Families* (Home Office/Ministerial Group on the Family 1998) also proposes measures to save salvageable marriages by enhanced access to marriage counselling. Whether these measures will reduce conflict in divorce, 'support' marriage and contain damage to children in the long run – and whether interventions are timed to take place at the right stage – remain to be seen. What is clear is that the private troubles for children caught up in divorce are now firmly on the public policy agenda.

Absent fathers

An even more controversial issue concerns the role of fathers in families, and the effects on children of growing up in a fatherless family. By the early 1990s, at least one father in seven was not living with any of his biological children (Burghes, Clarke and Cronin 1997, p. 65). Concerns about fatherless families arise in debates about family values, the role of fathers, and what is seen as a 'crisis in the family'.

Fatherless families

One prominent voice is that of Murray (Murray *et al.* 1990; Murray 1994) whose 'underclass' thesis has generated a great deal of controversy. Murray (Lister 1996, p. 25) describes the underclass in these terms:

> Britain has a growing population of working-aged, healthy people who live in a different world from other Britons, who are raising their children to live in it, and whose values are now contaminating the life of entire neighbourhoods.

In Murray's view the underclass can be defined through three characteristics: illegitimacy, lack of attachment to the labour market and violent, criminal behaviour. It has developed, he argues, partly because the stigma of illegitimacy has disappeared and welfare itself encourages people to have children outside marriage. Thus he suggests that many children are being born into fatherless families with no male role model, with disastrous social consequences. They in turn become irresponsible, optional and largely absent fathers incapable of the crucial role of socializing their children, particularly their sons, into a work ethic and a sense of community and family responsibility. As Halsey (in Dennis and Erdos 1993, p. xiv) puts it:

> [There is] an overlooked consequence of family breakdown – the emergence of a new type of young male, namely one who is both weakly socialized and weakly socially controlled so far as the responsibilities of spousehood and fatherhood are concerned.

This link asserted between 'contaminated values' and 'weak socialization' has contributed to the current emphasis in family policy on restoration of 'family values'. However, it is less clear what values these should be. Should family policies foster a conception of the father as a loving and authoritarian figure who is the main breadwinner and disciplinarian, as the traditional perspective favours (Dennis and Erdos 1993)? Or should they promote a more egalitarian model of active parenthood, with responsibilities of caring, socializing and breadwinning more equally shared between parents (Burgess and Ruxton 1998)?

Family policies and absent fathers

Family policies are not consistent in this respect. For example, the Child Support Act 1991 emphasizes the traditional financial responsibilities of (non-resident) fathers. But the Children Act 1989 and the Children (Scotland) Act 1995 adopt a more egalitarian perspective, seeing fathers as involved in a range of responsibilities towards their children. Of particular relevance to non-resident fathers are the legal rules governing parental rights of unmarried fathers, whether cohabiting or non-resident. The Children Acts of 1989 and 1995 introduced a concept of parental responsibility that pertains equally to fathers and mothers irrespective of marital status. Parental rights are seen as a means by which parents can fulfil their parental responsibilities. But married fathers have automatic parental rights while unmarried fathers must apply to a court for them (Burghes, Clarke and Cronin 1997). Few unmarried fathers seem aware of this, and it is not known whether lack of paternal rights has any practical effect (McRae 1993; Speak, Cameron and Gilroy 1997).

An egalitarian perspective might favour giving unmarried fathers equal status. This was considered by the Law Commission during the 1980s when abolishing the legal status of illegitimacy. However, objections were raised that this might not always be in the best interests of children. It would oblige a primary carer (usually the mother) to share decision-making with someone who previously may have had no responsibility for the child. It is not easy to identify the best interests of the child in a situation where parents are in conflict. Should the law oblige both parents to accept responsibility or give primary or even exclusive rights to one parent? Sevehuijsen (1989, p. 22) suggests that a 'primary care-take principle' – whereby the primary care-giver continues to care for children after partnership break-up – should be the basis for awarding custody, reducing the conflict associated with custody battles. Others advocate 'co-parenting' regardless of marital status. The Lord Chancellor has since proposed that unmarried fathers should automatically acquire equal parental rights.

Maintaining regular contact between children and their non-resident fathers (unless this is not in the child's interest) is seen as a desirable objective in the Children Act 1989 and the Children (Scotland) Act 1995. But other policies undermine this goal. The Child Support Act 1991 takes no account of the costs of travel or accommodation for children in the child support assessment formula (except in cases where these are especially large). Since it takes the financial obligation as primary, the impact of a child support assessment on the capacity to maintain contact is ignored. Moreover, local authority housing allocation policies give low priority to non-resident fathers so some will not have suitable accommodation for their children.

Deprivation and crime

While family policies may affect the involvement of fathers in socialization, the debate about fathers has focused more narrowly on the effects of absence. Much was made in the media (Phoenix 1996, p. 181) of a study (Dennis and Erdos 1993) suggesting that 'absent fatherhood' was connected with higher levels of delinquency and crime. This longitudinal study (of 264 men and women born in Newcastle in 1947) found that the families of children where the father had been continuously present were less likely to suffer multiple deprivation. It also found that men from families suffering multiple deprivation were much more likely to have criminal records.

Such associations between absent fatherhood, deprivation and crime are not straightforward. Deprivation indicators included 'general incompetence on the part of the mother' and 'poor physical and domestic care of the child' (requiring subjective judgements by researchers) along with more objective indicators such as debt and unemployment. 'Marital instability' was another indicator of deprivation, making the association between absent fatherhood and deprivation rather tautological. Moreover, very few fathers present in 'deprived' families were classed as 'good' or 'effective, kind and considerate' by the researchers – suggesting the presence of a father was insufficient to secure positive outcomes for children (Dennis and Erdos 1993, pp. 52–58). The debate on fatherless families tacitly implies that all is well where fathers are resident: a fixed gold standard. But is this so? Fatherhood generally is being transformed, although ideas are changing more rapidly than practice (Dench 1996). In Chapter 5 we consider more fully the contribution which fathers make to family life.

Non-resident need not mean uninvolved

Research suggests non-resident fathers are not necessarily absent, uninvolved, unsupportive or unavailable. A qualitative study of 40 young, non-resident fathers from disadvantaged backgrounds in Newcastle (Speak, Cameron and Gilroy 1997) found that they were committed to involvement with their children, and contributed in cash and in kind towards support of their child. They wanted to have greater contact with their children, but were prevented from doing so by barriers created by unemployment, inadequate income and lack of independent housing.

The large, complex and controversial body of research about the effects of non-resident fatherhood on children's development does suggest that children in fatherless households may suffer adverse outcomes. But the quality of the father/child relationship may be more important than the quantity of contact. Some of the negative consequences of fathers living apart from their children can be mitigated by a continuing good relationship between father and child and by a co-operative relationship between parents (Burghes, Clarke and Cronin 1997, pp. 69–70).

CONCLUSION

Although the role of families in socialization is increasingly shared with other social institutions, it occupies a pivotal focus for family policy. The British approach has tended to be non-interventionist, despite a slight shift in emphasis from 'problem families' to a general concern with how families socialize children. The focus on family 'problems' encourages a rather narrow preoccupation with family 'breakdown' and 'ineffective' parenting. These are legitimate concerns, but there is a danger in conceiving them within a problematic that seeks to blame rather than explain. Policies taking such a narrow view of issues of socialization, focusing on 'disrupted' or 'dysfunctional' families, may prove ineffective. Insofar as they promote a punitive perspective predicated on family pathology, they may add to the underlying pressures and problems which families experience and undermine the capacity of more vulnerable families to cope with their consequences. Family policy may be more usefully occupied with changing the conditions in which families socialize their children than with trying to change behaviour.

KEY POINTS

- Debates on socialization by families focus on whether its deficiencies are due to failures of parenting, unsatisfactory family forms, family disruption or the absence of fathers.
- Family policies on parenting have focused on interventions in problem families, tending towards non-intervention otherwise. This encourages a punitive preoccupation with family 'breakdown' and 'ineffective' parenting. Although effective parenting is a policy objective, identifying it is problematic. There is also a lack of agreement about policy objectives on sex education and prevention of teenage pregnancy.
- Family policies increasingly expect families, and especially parents, to support young people for a longer time as they make the transition to adulthood. Yet other policies have reduced families' resources. Many young people are not supported by their families, leaving them vulnerable to homelessness and unemployment.

- Evidence suggests that divorce and separation produce negative outcomes for children, including greater risks of educational, health and behaviour problems, and a greater chance of living in poverty and in poor housing. But poor outcomes may be caused by factors that occur before or at the time of divorce, rather than through divorce itself. Evidence also shows there is no inevitable link between family breakdown and negative outcomes for children, which may be mitigated by good parental relationships and minimizing parental conflict after divorce.
- Family policies that address the socialization role of fathers in families, and the potentially negative effects on children of growing up in a fatherless family include, for example, whether unmarried fathers should have equal parental rights and responsibilities. Research suggests non-resident fathers are not necessarily absent or unsupportive, and that associations between absent fatherhood, deprivation and crime are not straightforward.

GUIDE TO FURTHER READING

For details of children's changing living circumstances, see:

Clarke, L. (1996) 'Demographic change and the family situation of children' in Brannen, J. and O'Brien, M. (eds) (1996) *Children in Families: Research and Policy*, London: Falmer Press.

For details of parenting in the 1990s, see:

Ferri, E. and Smith, K. (1996) *Parenting in the 1990s*, London: Family Policy Studies Centre. (A summary appears as Findings No. 106, October 1996 at the Joseph Rowntree Foundation website.)

For a discussion of the effects of family breakdown and lone parenthood on children, see:

Burghes, L. (1994) *Lone parenthood and family disruption: the outcomes for children*, London: Family Policy Studies Centre.

For a review of research on divorce outcomes, see:

Rodgers, B. and Pryor, J. (1998) *Divorce and separation: the outcomes for children*, York: Joseph Rowntree Foundation. (A summary of both studies can be found at the Joseph Rowntree Foundation website – see Chapter 1).

For details of young people and family life, see:

Sweeting, H. and West, P. (1996) *The relationship between family life and young people's lifestyles,* Joseph Rowntree Foundation Findings No. 95 April 1996 (see website).

For traditionalist perspectives on fatherhood, see:

Murray, C., Field, F., Brown, J. C., Walker, A. and Deakin, N. (1990) *The Emerging British Underclass,* London: IEA.

Dennis, N. and Erdos, G. (1993) *Families without Fatherhood* (2nd ed), London: IEA.

For a review of research and policy on fatherhood, see:

Burghes, L., Clarke, L. and Cronin, N. (1997) *Fathers and fatherhood in Britain,* London: Family Policy Studies Centre.

For a policy perspective on fatherhood, see:

Burgess, A. and Ruxton, S. (1998) 'Men and their children' in Franklin, J. (ed.) (1998) *Social Policy and Social Justice,* Cambridge: Polity.

Care and Protection

4

Outline

In this chapter, we consider family policy in the context of family caring activities. Families are expected to provide care, and so it is important to recognize when they fail to do so. Such failures are not readily reconciled with the mythologies of the family which family policies tend to invoke. This is evident in the three issues discussed in this chapter, community care, child abuse and domestic violence, although in rather different ways. Policies to promote community care implicitly or explicitly rely on the caring role of families, particularly women. Child abuse challenges conceptions of the family as a caring institution and in particular our regard for its privacy. Responses to domestic violence tend to incorporate violence within a framework of (caring) family relationships assumed to render it less unacceptable – a matter for negotiation and management rather than prosecution. The effectiveness of policies which fail to distinguish rhetoric and reality is doubtful. It is especially difficult to strike an appropriate balance between the respective roles and responsibilities of family and state.

CARE IN FAMILIES

The routine business of care in families is supported by the state in many taken-for-granted ways. The NHS, still universal and mainly free on demand (especially where the health of children, people with disabilities and older people is concerned), supports the health-sustaining activities of families. Housing policies contribute (somewhat more selectively) to ensuring that families, by and large, can be adequately sheltered. Social rented housing has raised the housing standard of families with limited means, although it has been substantially weakened by privatization, deregulation and the withdrawal of housing subsidies.

The concept of 'care' as a form of work is a relatively new idea. It harbours overtones of expressing regard and assuming responsibility (as when we 'care for' or 'take care of' someone). But it has acquired a new resonance, as a set of activities (such as washing, cooking or dressing) to support those who for reasons of age or incapacity have particular needs. This has become a public concern mainly because of changing demographic and social trends, notably the growth of the 'elderly' population and the rising participation of women (the traditional 'carers') in paid employment. In the meantime feminist critiques of the gender division of labour have ensured that the question of 'Who cares?' has figured in policy debates.

CARING OBLIGATIONS AND INFORMAL CARE

The issue of 'Who cares?' raises many questions. One is the division between family and state over caring responsibilities. However this division is settled, the family will continue to provide care and other questions concern who shall or should provide it. The assumption that women will care has been weakened by changing expectations of their role in employment and their entitlements to leisure and personal fulfilment. Different assumptions may be made about the caring capacity of families in a population with diverse ethnic backgrounds. Moreover, caring may vary according to the age of the carer, as the problems of young carers may differ from those who are retired or approaching retirement.

From institutional care to community care

The issue of 'Who cares?' has been shaped by conceptions about where care should be given, and what care should be provided. Notable here is the shift to 'community care' and away from institutional forms of provision. Community care legislation, especially the National Health Service and Community Care Act 1990, shifted the emphasis from service provision by local authorities to a policy of 'enabling' provision through family and community. This created an internal market for community care, with local authorities purchasing care from a mixed economy of care providers drawn from the public, private, voluntary and informal sectors. This shift reflected a range of concerns, including financial pressures within the health and social services, as well as a growing emphasis on choice and independence for those requiring care. It has resulted in a greater privatization of care, on the assumption that the family will take on caring shed by the state.

This shift reflected a critique of institutional care, as an 'abnormal' social environment in which those who are cared for lacked power and choice – and were 'institutionalized' into dependence. This applied with particular force to 'asylums' for the mentally ill or handicapped, fuelled by a continuing succession of 'scandals' concerning the low standards of care and institutionalized violence against patients. For example, one report found sexual harassment of female patients rife in acute psychiatric wards in England and Wales, with problems including 'flashing', physical assaults and verbal harassment of vulnerable women (Ferriman 1997). Evidence that some 'patients' were confined for highly suspect motives reinforced the case against institutional provision. So too did an appreciation of the importance of a 'normal' environment for those in need of care, prompted in part by increasingly influential disability groups. The combined force of these criticisms led to a rapid run-down in some forms of institutional provision in favour of providing care in the more familiar environment of family and community.

In theory, the state in its 'enabling' role can offer more support to families to provide care and avoid unnecessary institutionalization. Doubts have been expressed, however, about the nature and extent of the support that has been offered. One criticism concerns the continuing gatekeeping role played by professional 'care managers' in community care, limiting autonomous decision-making by both carers and those who are cared for, despite the rhetoric of choice and empowerment attending the introduction of community care. Another criticism concerns the reluctance of governments to provide adequate financial support to those requiring care. In relation to long-term care for older people, the shift from health services provided in hospital to social care provided in the community has also involved a shift to means-testing. This has been especially controversial when it has required the sale of the family home to fund long-term care. In relation to disability, New Labour has also extended means-testing to reduce the cost of incapacity benefit. Lack of adequate funding to those requiring care may force them to depend on informal care – a dependency which may be less rather than more acceptable because of the strains it can impose upon the family.

Inequitable access to support is another important issue, not only in relation to gender (with male carers more likely to receive support) but also ethnicity. Ethnic groups may experience difficulties of access, partly related to language but also reflecting stereotypical assumptions about their inclination and capacity to provide care within the family without requiring further support. There is a dilemma in developing effective services for different ethnic groups, for absorption within mainstream provision may effectively marginalize support to ethnic groups, but so too may separate provision.

Informal care

Although informal care is unpaid, its economic value is substantial. In 1989 Britain's 6 million informal carers already provided about £20 billion of care. It is no exaggeration to say that the great majority of care for people with disabilities, long-term illnesses and for frail older people is provided by unpaid informal carers, usually within a family setting, and not by the private, voluntary or public sectors. The assumption that more care can be provided by families is questionable:

> The management and delivery of public care services for old people seem to be about to take real account of the contribution of the family just a moment too late, when the values that have made it care for its elderly are dissolving
>
> (Baldock 1993, p. 149)

Moreover, 'the level and quality of informal care in a community is not easily influenced, managed or bought' for it is the outcome of 'complex patterns of kinship, tradition and reciprocity' that develop in unpredictable ways (Baldock 1993, p. 147).

Caring responsibilities

A study by Finch and Mason (1993) examined how people acquire caring responsibilities. The authors undertook a quantitative study of 978 respondents in the Greater Manchester area, followed up by 120 interviews with a subset of respondents and their relatives. The research showed that people accept a general responsibility to support family members, which was seen as an unremarkable aspect of family life. It was more likely to be deemed acceptable, however, where the assistance required was limited in terms of time, effort and skill; where the need was perceived as genuine and legitimate; and where the relationship (most commonly parent/adult child) was sufficiently close to justify support.

Respondents saw caring less in terms of 'rights' and 'duties' than as a personal choice. Responsibilities were not so much inherited as created over time, through the accumulation of personal commitments and affiliations. Caring responsibilities were contingent and negotiated; more 'created commitments' than 'rules of obligation' (Finch and Mason, 1993, p. 173). People 'invested something of themselves' in certain relationships. Moral reputations could be undermined where claims for support were deemed undeserving or too unbalanced, leaving the cared-for person 'beholden' to the carer. Caring obligations were perceived as limited – a last and not a first resort. In general, people did not want to rely on relatives for extensive help, preferring 'intimacy at a distance' to an excessive sense of obligation to those closest to them.

It is ironic that the state should seek a residual caring role when families aspire to a similar role. As Finch and Mason comment:

> Policies which rest on the assumption that people have a right to expect assistance from their relatives ... will not align with the realities of family life. People do accept responsibilities to help relatives but ... want to retain the right ultimately to say that we do it of our own choosing.
>
> (Finch and Mason 1993, p. 180)

This point has now received partial recognition in the White Paper, *Caring about Carers*:

> the research emphasises that caring takes place within an existing relationship which is characterised by bonds of obligation, affection and reciprocity
>
> (DoH 1999, p. 23)

But it is difficult to distinguish the extent to which caring commitments result from an active choice or a more passive acceptance of 'duty' – some carers seem happy in a caring role while others find it grim. In similar vein, Twigg and Atkin (1994) distinguished carers 'engulfed' by caring (more likely women) from those (more likely men) achieving balance by setting boundaries and those positively benefiting from their caring role.

Gender, employment patterns and age of carers

Like many others Finch and Mason stressed the gender dimension of care as 'absolutely fundamental to the patterns of family responsibilities which most people develop in practice' (1993, p. 175). Because women are more likely to care for children and manage the home, they are more readily drawn into a web of reciprocal commitments. As commitments accumulate, women tend to become more firmly locked into caring roles. Ungerson (1987) in her study of carers also found that caring evolved through a history of personal relationships. But she argues that women are more prepared to accept caring as a 'duty':

> ... women, in contrast to men, are subject to considerable ideological and material pressure to be the carers of last resort, largely irrespective of their personal circumstances and whether or not as individuals they would rather spend their time in paid work or caring more completely for their children
>
> (Ungerson 1987, p. 83)

Nevertheless, informal care is not as obviously gendered as one might expect. The study *Informal Carers* estimates that there were 5.7 million carers in Britain in 1995: 3.3 million women (58%) and 2.4 million men (42%). There is an informal carer in one in six households, the great majority (90%) of whom care for a relative (DoH 1999, p. 17). Being a carer can mean a substantial time commitment, often involving a great deal of hard work and stress. About 30% of carers (1.7 million) provide 20 hours or more per week of care; half of these (855,000) provide over 50 hours. Men and women spend approximately the same amount of time providing care (DoH 1999, p. 18).

However, there are gender differences between carers. Men are most likely to be caring for their wives, whereas women are almost as likely to be caring for an elderly relative or a disabled child as for their husbands. Women are more likely than men to be the main carer (if there is more than one), and to provide care of a more intimate and urgent nature.

As one might expect, caring is related to employment patterns. Almost half (49%) of carers, and two-thirds of those below retirement age, are in paid employment; about one-quarter are retired (26%) or unemployed or economically inactive (25%). For many working carers, there are problems in reconciling their work and caring responsibilities (DoH 1999, p. 18).

Caring is also age-related, with a clear peak in the 45–64 age band, into which fall over two-fifths (41%) of all carers (DoH 1999, p. 18). The need to care tends to arise in middle age, when caring roles may be more acceptable as other commitments to childrearing or employment are complete. There are fewer expectations of young people to take on caring roles. Young carers may have to sacrifice other aspirations, such as schooling or friendships, especially when they take on heavy caring responsibilities while still in the education system.

Recognition of informal care

Thus informal care, even if available and acceptable, may involve much personal sacrifice for little reward, and conflict with other commitments such as schooling or employment. Yet recognition of informal carers in public policy is relatively recent, and largely due to feminist debates on community care. Limited recognition came in the Carers (Recognition and Services) Act 1995 intended to empower informal carers by giving them a voice and their needs a place in care planning and assessment. This recognition did not extend to giving carers resources to purchase support or alternative care themselves.

More recently, the National Strategy for Carers (DoH 1999) took account of research on informal caring, and at least pays lip service to the need for choice and voluntarism in care relationships:

> 10. We recognise that caring is founded on close relationships. The caring role grows out of the relationship and is one which most carers undertake from choice. Our objective is, therefore, focused on enabling those who choose to care, and whose care is wanted by another person, to do so without detriment to the carer's inclusion in society and to their health. Our aim is to support people who choose to be carers.
>
> 11. The Government's strategy for carers has three key approaches: Information for carers, so that they become real partners in the provision of the care to the person they are looking after, with the means to provide that care as well as they all wish to, and with wider and better sources of information about the help and services which are available to them. Support for carers, from the communities in which they live, in the planning and provision of the services that they and the person they are caring for use, and in the development of policies in the workplace which will help them to combine employment with caring. Care for carers, so that they can make real choices about the way they run their lives, so that they can maintain their health, exercise independence, and so that their role can be recognised by policymakers and the statutory services.
>
> (DoH 1999, pp. 13–14)

The National Strategy for Carers focuses on two groups of carers: young carers and carers in employment, and proposes a number of measures to help carers reconcile work and caring and improve support for carers. These include:

- personal advisors to help carers back into the labour market after caring

- a weekly addition to carers' pensions (up to £50 by 2050) to offset lost pension contributions
- mentors for young carers.

This approach is comprehensive, directed to many, and potentially all, families and having (at least some) explicitly stated policy goals. While the National Strategy for Carers is a path-breaking initiative, its importance may lie as much in changing attitudes as in the practical assistance it offers. The problems it addresses – how to improve the status and support of carers – are substantial and the resources allocated (£140 million) pale alongside the estimated £34 billion now saved through informal care. This may reflect its position that the family is the primary and leading partner in providing care and the state should take a secondary and supporting role.

Moreover, these first tentative steps towards supporting carers have to be considered in the context of policies towards those who are cared for. The disability movement has campaigned for provision of better financial support to recipients of care, to allow them to make independent choices about the care they require. It argues that the government has been reluctant – despite the rhetoric of empowerment of clients in community care – to offer financial support and give clients (rather than their care managers) a real choice in putting together packages of care.

Whether the idea of unequal partnership will differ significantly in practice from a residual safety net approach therefore remains to be seen. Much depends on related policies, such as state support for long-term care as recommended by the Royal Commission on Long Term Care in 1999. At the time of writing, initial responses of the Labour government suggested that the Commission's recommendation of free personal care paid for through general taxation was unlikely to be implemented.

CHILD PROTECTION

When care within families fails, society may act to protect vulnerable individuals. Family policies are typically couched in terms of support, empowerment and partnership between parents and the state. They may be perceived by families, however, in terms of regulation, control, and curtailment of parental preferences. It may be difficult, if not impossible, to support families as a whole while protecting vulnerable individuals within them.

Child abuse scandals demonstrate all too often the thorny dilemma of when the state, through social service departments, is justified in intervening in family life. The (public) childcare system acts in response to child neglect, physical or sexual abuse in families. The system operates through the courts (or Children's Panels in Scotland) and local authorities and other agencies responsible for substitute care for children. Child protection interventions reinforce (and sometimes even dictate) norms of family behaviour and define the boundaries between the family and the state, notably in judgements about the circumstances under which children can be involuntarily removed from their families.

The death of Maria Colwell in 1973 (Saraga 1993, p. 50) and further child deaths in the 1980s placed child abuse in the headlines and on the policy agenda. They focused attention on the effectiveness of social interventions to protect children from physical abuse. In the cases of Jasmine Beckford (1985), and of Tyra Henry and Kimberly Carlile (1987) social workers were castigated as 'excessive respecters of parental liberties' (Harding 1996, p. 164). Child sexual abuse again hit the headlines with the Cleveland scandal in 1987, and the Orkney inquiry in 1992 (Tisdall 1996). These focused on abuse within families but also on the procedures and practices of intervening agencies. Now, the social services were castigated for the converse offence of over-zealous interference in family life. While other higher status professions involved with children at risk of abuse – the police, doctors and teachers – may be given the benefit of the doubt, social workers tend to be criticized for neglect if they do not intervene and for interference if they do. Partly in response to these pressures, childcare interventions have increasingly focused on developing 'fail-safe' procedures for those children most at risk.

New statutes

Inquiries revealed the piecemeal nature of child protection, and encouraged a comprehensive review, culminating in the Children Act 1989 in England and Wales and the Children (Scotland) Act 1995 in Scotland. Both these statutes attempted to unify public and private childcare law and define a framework of parental rights and responsibilities. In keeping with the growing focus on the needs and rights of children, they also tried to establish the interests of children more securely by emphasizing the best interests of the child and ensuring that the child's voice is heard.

The Children Act 1989 set boundaries for intervention in family life by the state via the child protection system. In court proceedings, the child's welfare is regarded as paramount and decisions must take account of children's wishes. The Act established rights for children to representation in court, to make formal complaints, to challenge the decisions of local authorities to seek an Emergency Protection Order or Child Assessment Order, and, in limited circumstances, to seek a Contact or Residence Order to determine with whom they should have contact and where they should live.

The Act also defined the concept of parental responsibility as a set of duties, rights and authority. Parental responsibility is accorded primary status, in the belief that children are cared for best within the family without outside intervention in the form of legal proceedings. The courts should not take action unless intervention is clearly better for the child than not intervening. The Act assumes that children's welfare may be best served by giving support to their parents. The primacy of parental responsibility (which remains even when children are receiving substitute care) is reinforced by the language of the 1989 Act. Thus children are said to be 'looked after' by local authorities, rather than 'in care'. If a child is receiving substitute care, local authorities must try, whenever possible, to maintain family contact. This takes account of research findings that showed the importance of contact for future planning and returning home (Hill and Aldgate 1996). It is also recognizes that parents should be able to seek help without risking an unwarranted response on the part of childcare authorities:

> It was seen as important that families should be able to seek help for everyday difficulties in parenting, without undue fears of a draconian response
>
> (Hill and Aldgate 1996, p. 5)

There is therefore an emphasis on partnership with parents, evident in the requirement to consult parents and seek their consent in decisions relating to the child's future. The Act thus tries to achieve a balance between child protection and family support, in tacit recognition of the close association between child abuse and neglect and families under stress. In Harding's view:

> [the Children Act 1989] tried to protect family autonomy and give parents *more* rights by making the emergency provisions for removing children less weighted against the parents ... The bias

> was towards letting families/parents sort out their own disputes and difficulties ... [The Act] appears to support and maintain original family units rather than enhance the compulsory powers of the state to separate parents and children
>
> (Harding 1996, pp. 164–165)

On the other hand, if the court does make an order, this can have a profound impact on the family involved. Parental rights and responsibilities can still be suspended, parents can be prevented from seeing their children, and in some cases, children can be adopted without parental consent.

While the 1989 Act made the interests of children paramount, it also emphasized the roles and rights of parents and set children's rights within a broadly legalistic setting. By contrast, The Children Act (Scotland) 1995, in the context of a more 'child-friendly' Children's Panel system, established a broader duty to take account of the views of a child (so far as practicable) on any decisions by those exercising parental responsibility on their behalf.

A balancing act

Whatever the legislative balance, social workers and other professionals continue to face difficult choices in trying to reconcile the potentially conflicting interests of children and their parents. Although the legislation aims to give children a voice, it may not be heard, especially if procedures remain legalistic and professionals remain under severe pressure arising from risk of media condemnation.

The general framework set out under this legislation seems likely to persist, but the emphasis on managing risk suggests a need for more family support to prevent abuse in the first place. In *Supporting Families* (Home Office/Ministerial Group on the Family 1998), there is a proposal to create Parentline, a national parent helpline service for information and referral to local sources of help, based on Childline. The Consultation Paper, *Working Together to Safeguard Children: New Government Proposals for Inter-agency Co-operation* states in its preface:

> Ensuring that all children within our community are safeguarded and protected from abuse is an objective to which the Government is firmly committed. We believe that the community as a whole has a responsibility for promoting the welfare of children and for the prevention of child abuse and neglect. Families provide the prime building block for safe and sustainable communities and all agencies and professionals need to support parents in discharging

> their parental rights and responsibilities to enhance the welfare and safety of children ... We need to take a wider, more holistic view of the needs of vulnerable children and their families ... We know that many of the families who find themselves caught up in the child protection system suffer from multiple disadvantages. They need help at an earlier stage to tackle their problems before parenting difficulties escalate into abuse ... However, the Government recognises that an effective child protection system will continue to be needed to deal with cases of abuse.
>
> (DoH 1998, p. 1)

This accepts that greater family support may have a critical role to play in child protection:

> the current emphasis on individual risk strategies in the prevention of child abuse and neglect, and in the protection of children from harm, has to change
>
> (Spencer 1996, p. 154).

However, as always in family policy there may some distance between general rhetoric and the limited reality of policies to provide the needed support. Child protection policies would have to be allied with a raft of other measures to improve the capacity of families to cope with conflict, sustain living standards and reconcile the competing demands of home and work.

DOMESTIC VIOLENCE AND FAMILY POLICY

Care and protection in families also fails when domestic violence occurs between adults. This refers mainly to violence between spouses, cohabitees and separated partners. Since domestic violence reached the public policy agenda in the early 1970s, violence between partners has become recognized as a common feature of family life. Its measurement is difficult, as violence is often hidden or unreported, and definitions vary. Nevertheless research suggests that domestic violence is extensive, and can be frequent and severe (Morley and Mullender 1994).

Incidence of domestic violence

An early study of Scottish police statistics found one-third of all violent offences (and the majority of all violent offences where the victim was female) were domestic in origin; 70% of these incidents consisted of violence by husbands on wives (Dobash and Dobash 1979). Domestic violence is the most common violent crime against women in England and Wales, with about 835,000 incidents reported in 1997 (Home Office/Ministerial Group on the Family 1998, p. 45), representing nearly half of all violent offences against women (Home Office 1999). Because of high levels of underreporting and underrecording, these figures underestimate the incidence of domestic violence.

The 1996 British Crime Survey (Mirrlees-Black 1998) of a nationally representative sample of over 10,000 people in England and Wales aged 16–59 found that 4.9% of men and 5.9% of women reported assault or threats by a partner in the last year. Women were more likely to suffer injury and repeated assaults. One-quarter of women (26%) and 17% of men had suffered such violence in the past, with women again more likely to suffer repeated assaults. Asked about the most recent violence, respondents reported incidents such as being kicked, slapped, punched, having things thrown at them, and less often: choking, strangling, suffocating or being raped. Most of these incidents (53%) were not reported to anyone; only 11% were reported to the police.

Half of those reporting violence in the previous year were living with children, of whom 29% had witnessed the violence. Children were even more likely to witness violence when it was recurrent. Other research shows that violence against a partner is commonly associated with child abuse or neglect – in 60% of cases where children suffer neglect, physical or emotional abuse, mothers were also subject to abuse from their male partners (Home Office/Ministerial Group on the Family 1998, p. 45).

Explanations and responses

There are many competing explanations for domestic violence, including psychological explanations of stress, psychoanalytic and family systems therapeutic theories, individual pathologies (of both perpetrator and victim), sociological explanations based on deprivation factors, and feminist analyses of male power (Dobash and Dobash 1992; Dallos and McLaughlin 1993). These explanations often implicitly inform the different rationales put forward to justify the intervention of the state into 'private troubles' of families, and these rationales sometimes clash.

Ideas about the protection of vulnerable family members underlie many of the remedies found in family law. From a traditional perspective, the state ought not interfere in family life unless something has gone wrong. The difficulty here is in determining when abuse goes beyond the normal wear and tear of marriage, rendering an individual 'vulnerable' and warranting intervention. Competing with this conditional basis for intervention is another based on citizenship, and civil rights (and informing criminal law): that any individual has a right to expect protection from the state from physical assault, wherever it takes place.

Domestic violence thus raises questions about the role of the state in the private sphere of the family and challenges established boundaries between public and private life. Responses to domestic violence range across several areas of government activity and have various objectives, from protection and service provision for victims to punishment and social control of offenders and regulation of intimate relationships. Taken as a whole, they exemplify policies targeted selectively towards 'problem families', with implicit and often contradictory policy objectives and underlying assumptions.

Policies on domestic violence

There have been numerous policies relating to domestic violence, as the issue itself has waxed and waned on the public policy agenda since the 1970s. These have developed in a climate of social change including the maturing of feminism, the growth of a grass-roots refuge movement and an increasing recognition that domestic violence is a legitimate issue for policies to address. There are more than 250 Women's Aid groups operating over 400 refuges in England and Wales (Women's Aid Federation of England 1996; Home Office 1999) – providing temporary, safe, emergency accommodation for 50,000 women and children during 1994–1995 (WAFE Annual Survey, 1995). Nevertheless the continuing demand for refuge space is evidence that this 'private trouble' shows no sign of disappearing.

In recent years efforts have been made to produce co-ordinated responses, at least if measured by the creation of administrative structures. An Interdepartmental Working Party on Domestic Violence was set up in 1994. This was followed by a Ministerial Group and an Interdepartmental Official Group on Domestic Violence to co-ordinate government action in this area. In 1997 two Ministers for Women were appointed, with a supporting Women's Unit within the Cabinet Office. A Scottish Partnership on Domestic Violence was set up in 1998 and a Domestic Violence Forum in Northern Ireland (Home Office 1999). The government recently announced that 'Tackling domestic violence is a crucial part of our family policy' (Home Office/Ministerial Group on the Family 1998, p. 45). The measures mentioned in *Supporting Families* (Home Office/Ministerial Group on the Family 1998, p. 40) consist of:

> better reporting, a tougher attitude by the police and courts, the first national survey of refuges for survivors of violence and a new national publicity campaign.

In July 1999 the government followed this up with further measures, including an increased grant to Victim Support and a proposed 24-hour helpline.

Nevertheless, developments in civil law, policing, social work practice and housing reflect the fragmented, dispersed nature of policies addressing the failure of care and protection in families – and the lack of a comprehensive or coherent policy approach overall.

Civil law remedies

In civil law, section IV of the Family Law Act 1996 (for England and Wales) consolidated previous law on domestic violence and established court orders to give specific protection for its victims. For example, an occupation order gives one partner a right to occupy the family home and can exclude a partner. Where violence or a threat of violence has already occurred, a power of arrest may be attached to a non-molestation order. These orders can apply to spouses, cohabitees or former spouses or cohabitees for a limited period. Some protection is afforded to cohabitees from domestic violence (for example, for transfers of tenancy), but their status in relation to spouses is inferior because they lack the original commitment of marriage.

Moreover, other changes to the legal system – notably the changes making access to civil legal aid more restrictive – may reduce women's access to justice and prevent them from using the remedies available to them.

Criminal law and the police

The police provide the only 24-hour emergency protection from domestic violence in all areas, so this is the public agency most commonly contacted by victims. However, the police have traditionally been reluctant to intervene in 'domestic disputes' between husbands and wives, and their support has received consistent negative evaluations by victims. Research has shown repeatedly that police define the problem as one they are not empowered to deal with, do not regard domestic violence as a crime, underreport such incidents, and seldom arrest assailants (Morley and Mullender 1994, p. 13). Pressure for a more sympathetic and responsive police service has included calls for greater use of arrest, and a more co-ordinated response among agencies within the criminal justice system (police, prosecutors and courts) and other social and community services.

Policies introduced from the late 1980s required police to reassess their practices and attitudes. A Home Office Circular in 1990 signalled that domestic violence is a criminal offence, that assailants are responsible for their acts and that the police should protect and empower victims. Recommendations included a reminder that the criminal law gave police the power and the duty to take positive action on domestic violence, including arrest; that it was not their job to mediate; and that they should take steps to support and minimize the risk of harm to the victim. The circular also recommended more systematic recording of offences and establishment of domestic violence units.

By 1991, policy statements on domestic violence had been adopted by all police forces in England and Wales (Morley and Mullender 1994, p. 17). There have also been institutional changes. Many forces established dedicated Domestic Violence Units to co-ordinate agency responses, to provide a more experienced and specialized service, and monitor and improve general attitudes and practice. These received generally favourable evaluations from both victims and advocacy groups (Morley and Mullender 1994, p. 18). Some police forces also take an active part in Domestic Violence Forums that co-ordinate the response of different agencies at a local level. Whether these institutional changes have produced the desired degree of change in police practice nationally is not known, but early evidence suggests there have been some improvements in practice in many, but not all, areas. However, Domestic Violence Units may marginalize domestic violence from mainstream policing. Policies have focused on offering a better service to the victims of domestic violence, without parallel policies to change attitudes and challenge the behaviour of its perpetrators.

Housing and local authority practice

Housing has an important role to play to give women and children escaping domestic violence somewhere safe to go. Since the 1970s, housing policies and housing agency practice in some areas have recognized that role to a limited extent, principally by:

- providing property and funding for refuges run by Women's Aid and other voluntary organizations
- accepting families escaping from domestic violence as homeless and in need of permanent re-housing
- modifying allocation rules to give priority for re-housing and tenancy transfers to families escaping domestic violence.

Tackling domestic violence (Cabinet Office 1998) considers how local authorities have dealt with domestic violence, especially in terms of support for victims, and partnerships with the police and other organizations. It presents evidence of good practice but also of patchy coverage and inadequate funding, based on returns from 30% of local authorities. Over 200 Domestic Violence Forums, typically including the police, women's aid groups and other statutory and voluntary bodies, had been set up by 1996. These were the main vehicle for inter-agency work on domestic violence. The range of activities varied widely, from examples of changing practices in the criminal courts and the police to public awareness campaigns.

A smaller proportion of local authorities (one in six) also reported they had a corporate policy on domestic violence, with a member of staff with responsibility for co-ordinating work on domestic violence. However, funding for work on domestic violence varied greatly and was often insecure and fragmented where it did exist. Women's Aid was a focus for local activity on domestic violence, but much depended on voluntary effort, funding for refuges was inadequate and refuge provision did not exist everywhere it was needed.

These examples of family policy operating at a local level show how it can give scope for innovation and good practice, but can result in fragmented policy making, and patchy coverage.

CONCLUSION

This chapter considered three case studies of family policies linked to the activities of care and protection. Community care is an explicit family policy that states the conditions under which state interventions in family life will be made. While informed by research on informal carers, it has not taken on board all its lessons. Community care policy is at odds with evidence that those who need and those who might offer care in families want choice and often see the family as a last resort and not a first resort. Although we often equate the 'family' with the 'private' and the state with the 'public' sphere, public policies shape family life and construct a particular set of familial social relations. In this case, policy is normative, i.e. it suggests what familial caring obligations ought to be and what will be reinforced and supported. It presumes that the family setting is the preferred location for community care, and that primary care is best delivered by family members. Policies which shift responsibility to families for providing care may have adverse implications for those supposed to meet these obligations. Family policies have only begun to address these issues.

The policies that have emerged in response to child abuse and domestic violence have sometimes had explicit broad objectives to 'tackle' the problem. However, they have tended to express a 'problem family' orientation that is directed to responding to or reducing recurrences of violence or abuse. This approach has underplayed policies directed towards prevention of abuse or violence or towards enforcing the rights of victims. Existing policies span a wide range of government activities, and operate at both national and local levels. With regard to child abuse, policies have become more child focused, but with a new emphasis too on 'partnership' with parents, and a continuing reluctance to take a preventive rather than remedial approach.

Policies on domestic violence have lacked coherence, been partial in coverage, and have often been *ad hoc*. The 'modest and reluctant' approach to this issue that is typical of so much of family policy in Britain has produced insecure and inadequate resourcing of programmes focusing on domestic violence. How far this is now changing remains to be seen. Policies to tackle the underlying causes of family violence and abuse have hardly been considered.

KEY POINTS

- Community care policies rely on families, particularly women, assuming a major caring role. Gender is fundamental to understanding care provided by families. Most care for frail older people, people with disabilities and long-term illnesses is already provided by informal carers within the family, and not by the private, voluntary or public sectors. An ageing population will increase demand for informal care while the supply of traditional 'carers' will fall due to women's greater participation in paid employment.
- The policy assumption that more care can be provided by families is questioned by research showing that caring responsibilities in families are more 'created commitments' than 'rules of obligation'. Although the state in its 'enabling' role can support families who provide care, doubts exist about that support. Recent recognition of informal carers in public policy is seen in proposals to improve their status and the support available.
- Policies on domestic violence and child protection raise questions about when and how the state is justified in intervening in family life, and challenge boundaries between public and private spheres.
- Child protection policies have a 'problem family' focus and aim to strike a balance between child protection, parental responsibility and family support.
- Domestic violence is recognized as a widespread example of where families' protection activities fail. Policy responses to domestic violence, in policing, civil law, social work and housing, have objectives of protection and services for victims and punishment and control of offenders but have been fragmented, modest, *ad hoc* and targeted towards 'problem families'.

GUIDE TO FURTHER READING

For an introductory discussion of the role of informal carers in community care, see:

Ungerson, C. (1998) 'The Informal Sector' in Alcock, P., Erskine, A. and May, M. (eds) (1998) *The Student's Companion to Social Policy*, Oxford: Blackwell and the Social Policy Association.

For a qualitative study on family obligation that raises questions for community care policies, see:

Finch, J. and Mason, J. (1993) *Negotiating Family Responsibilities,* London: Tavistock/Routledge.

For further discussion of child protection and family policy, see:

Daniel, P. and Ivatts, J. (1998) *Children and Social Policy,* Basingstoke, Macmillan.

Harding, L. (1997) *Perspectives in Child Care Policy* (Second edition), London: Longman.

and the edited collection:

Hill, M. and Aldgate, J. (eds) (1996) *Child Welfare Services: Developments in law, policy, practice and research,* London: Jessica Kingsley. (Especially the chapters by Hill and Aldgate on the Children Act 1989 and the chapter by Tisdall on the Children (Scotland) Act 1995.)

For a review of policy responses to domestic violence in the 1980s and early 1990s, see:

Dobash, R. E. and Dobash, R. P. (1992) *Women, Violence and Social Change,* London: Routledge.

For a review of literature on domestic violence, see:

Morley, R. and Mullender, A. (1994) *Preventing Domestic Violence to Women,* Home Office CPU Paper 48, London: Home Office.

For a recent survey on the incidence of domestic violence. see:

Mirrlees-Black, C. (1998) *Domestic Violence: findings from a new British Crime Survey self-completion questionnaire: Home Office Research Study No. 192,* London: Home Office.

Family income and resource distribution

5

Outline

With growing poverty and inequality in British society, how resources are transferred between and within families has become an important issue for family policy. In this chapter we discuss both vertical distribution (from well-off to poor families) and horizontal distribution (between families in different circumstances). Like its predecessors, the Labour government is increasingly inclined to define family policies in terms of vertical distribution – to target resources on those families 'most in need'. In contrast, the rights-based agenda which informs universal benefits such as Child Benefit has been marginalized. The problem of reducing dependency by increasing work incentives has also loomed large, obscuring issues concerned with the needs of families for an adequate standard of living. Issues of poverty raise questions about how resources are transferred within families, including women's rights to independent income. The shift from a rights-based approach to concerns with responsibility is nowhere more evident than in the introduction of the Child Support Act, which provides a text-book example of the difficulties of translating simple principles into effective practice.

THE ECONOMICS OF FAMILY LIFE

Families involve economic as well as social and emotional bonds. Families can even be considered mainly as media of economic exchange. Some economists analyse family transactions in terms of economic calculations; some feminists have seen marriage as a trade-off of economic support for sexual satisfactions. Living in families has implications for how resources are transferred, distributed and consumed.

Living together as a family may have economic benefits, through sharing income and housing costs. Families also share food, transport, entertainment and other aspects of everyday life. They share the costs of child-rearing. Through sharing and specialization, families can achieve improvements in their standards of living (Papps 1980, p. 16). How should such 'economies' be valued when providing families with financial support?

Families also entail additional costs. Direct costs may include anything from televisions to mobile phones. We must also consider opportunity costs, particularly for parents (usually mothers) taking time out from employment to raise children. One estimate put the average cost of a child (to age 17) at £50,000 – 90% of which is met by parents (Middleton *et al.* 1997). The costs of supporting other family members (perhaps unemployed or disabled) must also be considered.

How far should society meet, mitigate or redistribute the costs which families incur? Should policies seek redistribution of costs between families or over their life-cycle? Should family policies redistribute resources from richer to poorer families (vertical redistribution)? Should family policies redistribute resources from households without children to those with children (horizontal redistribution)? How adequate are resource transfers (such as tax rebates and social security benefits) for meeting the needs of families who receive them? Should parents meet the costs of children who no longer live with them? Can society ensure that people fulfil their obligations to current or former partners and children? Such questions have acquired a greater urgency given the increase in the number of children living in poverty, the growing inequality between households with and without children, and the growth of divorce, lone-parent families and stepfamilies.

Policies make inconsistent assumptions about the extent of family resource transfers. In assessing Income Support, it is assumed that an adult with a spouse and dependent children should be treated as a single benefit unit within which income is shared. Non-dependent adults within the household (such as a grandparent or young adult not in full-time education) are treated as separate benefit units where income is not shared. Housing Benefit assumes that non-dependent adults in the household contribute to housing costs, and benefit is calculated accordingly. In contrast, Child Benefit is paid directly to the primary carer assuming that income sharing is limited.

Fiscal pressures have prompted government to redraw the boundaries of family and state responsibility, notably regarding support for young people, and the obligations of 'absent' parents. Taxation and other policies increasingly assess individuals independently, reflecting a general shift to recognizing the rights and responsibilities of individuals within family units.

ADEQUACY OF RESOURCES

Family and child poverty has increased sharply. Between 1979 and the mid-1990s, the proportion of children in households with incomes below half of the national average rose from 9% to 34% (DSS 1998a). The median income of the poorest 10% of households fell by 5%, while average incomes rose by over 40%. The proportion of lone parents in the bottom fifth of income distribution grew from 9% in 1979 to 24% in 1995/1996. Do social security benefits provide adequate support for these families?

Assessments of adequacy have calculated the costs of raising children for different 'model' families by costing a given 'basket of goods' compared to income from scale rates (Table 5.1).

Table 5.1 A comparison of the Modest But Adequate (MBA) budget with Income Support (£ per week, 1995 prices)

	Lone mother + two young children	Couple + two young children
Total MBA less housing costs	281.69	250.25
Income support	93.85	115.15
% of MBA budget met by income support	33%	46%

Source: Oppenheim and Harker (1996) (derived from Modest But Adequate: summary budgets for sixteen households, Family Budget Unit 1995)

A Modest But Adequate budget 'represents a level of income which allows people to participate fully in society rather than simply exist' (Oppenheim and Harker 1996, p. 42). It includes:

- £6.25 for alcohol, but nothing for tobacco
- 1 week's annual holiday, but not abroad.

A more stringent budget (Table 5.2) can be derived by eliminating or reducing spending on various items (such as alcohol).

Table 5.2 Comparison of the low-cost budgets and the Income Support rate for two adult/two child and one adult/two child families (April 1993 prices, £ per week)

	1 adult/2 child	2 adult/2 child
Total low-cost budget (LCB)	111.73	142.56
Income support (IS)	88.65	108.75
% of LCB budget met by IS	78%	76%

Source: Derived from Oldfield and Autumn (1993) Table 24 p. 56

The researchers concluded that 'although the low cost budgets are fairly stringent, Income Support rates do not allow the families with children to reach even a low cost standard of living' (Oldfield and Autumn 1993, p. 56). Using survey data showing how much money families need, Berthoud and Ford (1996) also found that the 'true' costs of children were much more than the sums allowed in any of the social security scale rates for children.

Scale rates take account of the age of children and their place in the family. Income Support and the new Working Families Tax Credit (Table 5.3) differentiate by the age of a child. Studies do not altogether support these assumptions. Berthoud and Ford found that the cost of children did not rise as children became older. They did, however, find that the cost of the first child exceeded the costs of subsequent children – consistent with Child Benefit, which has a higher rate for the first child. Using Family Expenditure Survey data, Dickens, Fry and Pashardes (1995) found that the costs of the first and second child were greater than subsequent children, while lone-parent families had much higher relative costs than two-parent families. However, the greater costs of lone-parent families have been discounted by governments determined to remove additional benefit premiums for lone parents.

Making ends meet

Adequacy can also be assessed by investigating how families cope. Can they 'make ends meet'? A review of research suggests many families cannot (Kempson 1996). A study of 200 lone-parent families in Greater London during 1992/1993 found that no matter how positive parents were about shopping for 'healthy' foods, those with lower incomes had less healthy diets than better-off families. Parents tended to go without rather than let their children suffer (Dowler and Calvert 1995). Studies of families on low incomes present a bleak picture of struggling to survive through a variety of strategies:

- shopping little and often to avoid stocks being eaten
- searching systematically for special offers
- shopping alone (to reduce pressures from children)
- using convenience foods to avoid waste
- buying foods with high fat/sugar contents to meet immediate needs.

People go without essentials, juggle bills or use credit to get by. Kempson suggests that only a minority of families with children can keep their heads above water over the long-term. A 1993 survey of lone parents found three-quarters had debts over the preceding 3 years, with a third often in debt (Ford *et al.* 1995, p. 30). Oppenheim and Harker (1996, p. 75) report that many Income Support claimants live below the basic benefit level because of deductions for arrears.

Reviewing all the available evidence, Kempson concluded that unless they had other resources to draw on, families living on social security could not make ends meet. Other resources could be significant:

> Most people who lived on low incomes received financial help and support from friends and family. And the poorer they were, the more they relied on them for necessities. There was also a great deal of reciprocity, with people helping one another out as and when they could.
>
> (Kempson 1996, p. 57)

But help was acceptable only within limits:

> ... people clearly found some types of help more acceptable than others. Help in kind was considered better than cash, and loans were better than gifts – especially gifts of cash, which were seen as charity and to be avoided wherever possible. Being able to reciprocate in some way was essential to maintaining dignity.
>
> (Kempson 1996, p. 59)

Obliging people to rely on such sources cannot guarantee their living standards, and may undermine their sense of moral worth.

Policy options

How should the state support low family incomes? The government stresses the importance of employment as 'the best route out of poverty for those who can work' (DSS 1998d, p. 19). It intends to shift state support for low-income families from out-of-work benefits to in-work benefit top-ups to low wages: 'The Government's aim is to rebuild the welfare state around work' (DSS 1998d, p. 23). The New Deal involves state support in helping people find work, more education, training, childcare and other incentives and subsidies to employers. The aim is to make it more financially attractive for families to be in work than on Income Support.

The principal benefit for low-income working families with children will be the Working Families Tax Credit (WFTC), which replaced Family Credit in October 1999. Working Families Tax Credit is set at a more generous level and gives more recognition to formal childcare costs. It is withdrawn more gradually as income rises above a threshold of £90 (deducted at 55p for each £1 of net income rather than 70p). It aims to reduce the poverty trap which leaves families financially worse off in work than on benefit because of the loss of housing benefit and tax and national insurance contributions deducted from income.

The benefit includes a basic rate plus scale rates for children that increase with the child's age (Table 5.3).

Table 5.3 Structure of Working Families Tax Credit (£ per week, 1998–1999 prices)

Basic tax credit (one payable per family)		48.40
Tax credits for each child aged	0–11	14.85
	11–16	20.45
	16–18	25.40
30 hours tax credit		10.80
Taper (amount withdrawn as % of every additional £1 of net income over threshold)		55p

Source: HM Treasury (1998) *The Modernisation of Britain's Tax and Benefit System Number Three: The Working Families Tax Credit and work incentives*, p. 9.

However, concerns remain over whether WFTC will have the intended impact on family poverty, partly because of doubts that it will make a significant difference to the poverty trap of families (Family Policy Studies Centre 1998a). Critics argue that as WFTC is means-tested it will encourage employers to set minimum wage levels and employees to accept them. Since Family Credit was usually paid to the woman and WFTC may be paid to the man (Goode, Callender and Lister 1998) there is also concern over which parent receives the tax credit and its effect on distribution of income *within* families.

EQUITY AND CHILD BENEFIT

As well as adequacy, issues of equity are important in family policy. On average, families with children have lower incomes than those without, and two-parent families are much better off than lone-parent families. The average gross income in 1994/1995 of couples (below retirement age) without children was £499 per week; the corresponding figure for couples with children was £460 per week, and lone-parent families £190 per week (Family Policy Studies Centre 1998a). Family Allowances were designed to achieve greater fairness by redistributing incomes to families with children from those without, since even with similar resources, families with children are generally thought to have greater needs. It also transferred income to periods of child-rearing from periods without. It was replaced in 1977 by Child Benefit, which also incorporated tax allowances for children.

Child Benefit is a tax-free benefit paid directly to the principal carer (usually the mother) for every child up to the age of 16, and up to the age of 19 for those who are unmarried and in full-time secondary education. It is a universal benefit – not based on previous contributions or means-testing. Almost all those eligible actually claim and receive it – about 7 million families and 12.5 million children at a cost of £6.5 billion in 1996/1997 (DSS 1998b, p. 6).

The state has accepted only limited responsibility to help families with children. Family allowances were 'intended to assist with (but not wholly absorb) the additional expense of bringing up children' (Henwood and Wicks 1986, p. 11). The value of Child Benefit has always been well short of the costs of a child – one-fifth of average costs in one estimate (Middleton *et al.* 1997). By the mid-1990s it was worth less to most families than the system it replaced.

Thus the main means of equalizing incomes between families with and without children has been substantially eroded. This reflects a growing preoccupation with poverty rather than equity. Governments have preferred means-tested anti-poverty measures such as Family Credit and the Working Families Tax Credit. It also reflects the decline in a collective commitment to reproduction. While Beveridge in the 1940s believed (with eugenic overtones) that 'housewives as mothers have vital work to do in ensuring the adequate continuance of the British race and of British ideals in the world'; by the Meade Commission of 1978 children had become 'an expensive hobby' (Henwood and Wicks 1986, p. 7). As a result, attention has shifted from horizontal redistribution (between families with and without children) to vertical distribution (from better-off families to those most in need).

Is Child Benefit secure under the present government? The government puts its view thus:

> Child Benefit remains the fairest, most efficient and cost effective way that society can recognise the extra costs and responsibilities borne by all parents. So Child Benefit, which is society's support for, and investment in, the upbringing of children, should be available to all. We made this a commitment in our manifesto where we said that we would 'retain universal Child Benefit where it is universal today – from birth to age 16 – and uprate it at least in line with prices' ... If Child Benefit were raised in future, there must be a case in principle for higher tax payers paying tax on it. The Government wants to move from general support to all couples to particular support for couples with children, so the Child Benefit increase will be paid for by reducing the value of the married couple's and associated allowances.
>
> (Home Office/Ministerial Group on the Family 1998, p. 20)

This is a rather ambivalent endorsement of the only universal support available to families with children in the UK. The lack of a commitment to link increases in Child Benefit to earnings rather than prices implies its steady erosion as a significant method of horizontal redistribution to those families with children.

In the March 1999 Budget, Child Benefit was increased at more than the rate of inflation, to £15 per week for a first child and £10 per week for other children from April 2000. Despite these increases, Labour seems to see Child Benefit mainly as a passive and inequitable method of family support. Hence much mooted proposals to tax the Child Benefit of those on the highest rate of income tax, or to switch Child Benefit for 16–18 year olds to funding for Educational Maintenance Allowances (EMAs) targeted on lower-income families (Treasury 1999, p. 36). The married couples tax allowance will be replaced from 2001 by a new children's tax credit tapered away from higher earning families.

However, a problem with measures to target family support more selectively is that they can involve high marginal tax rates (that can reach as high as 96p in £1) as benefit is withdrawn as income increases (and taxes also rise). Thus selective transfers may target those most in need but do so in ways that may create disincentives to work. Critics of the selective approach argue that Child Benefit is an important independent income source to all mothers, most especially with low incomes, and is seen as being for their children (Goode, Callender and Lister 1998, p. 10; Bradshaw and Stimson 1997).

THE CASE OF CHILD SUPPORT

As well as transferring resources between families, policies can affect transfers within them. This was the aim of the Child Support Act 1991, if we allow that 'families' include non-resident parents. It enforced a child's right to support from both biological parents, irrespective of their legal relationship (married or not) and whether they lived with the child. It was prompted by the rapid growth in the number of lone parents and a decline in the maintenance payments they received. Growth in public expenditure on lone parents (£2.4 billion in 1978/1979 to £6.6 billion in 1992/1993) was a major factor. Underpinning reform was a concern about 'family values', illustrated by Margaret Thatcher's 1990 statement to the 300 Group:

> Government too must be concerned to see parents accept responsibility for their children. For even though marriages may break down, parenthood is for life. Legislation cannot make irresponsible parents responsible. But it can and must ensure that absent parents pay maintenance for their children. It is not fair for them to expect other families to foot their bills too

This view gained much public support. The Child Support Act set up the Child Support Agency (CSA) for all child support assessment, collection and enforcement. Assessment was removed from the courts and calculated by a standard but complex formula. It became compulsory for all parents with care receiving Income Support and Family Credit, although optional for others.

Implementation of the Act proved unpopular, expensive and

ineffective – a major policy failure of the 1990s. High savings targets have produced few winners among absent parents and parents with care. Compliance has been poor; in 1997 two-thirds of those on Income Support did not wish to apply for maintenance, despite risking a benefit penalty (Home Office/Ministerial Group on the Family 1998, p. 22). Procedures were overly complex and lengthy, with errors, backlogs and delays in collection common. One-third of assessments took more than 6 months to complete, and two-fifths of assessments involved errors (DSS 1998c). The sums collected and transferred to children were far less than under the previous system; in 1993/1994, only £15 million was paid through the CSA, compared with over £200 million through previous arrangements in 1992/1993 (DSS 1998c).

Under the 1991 Act, those lone parents (mainly mothers) most in need of maintenance are least likely to receive it. For lone parents on Income Support, maintenance payments are deducted pound for pound from their benefit entitlement. If payments are sufficiently high to lift a mother off Income Support, she may lose entitlement to 'passported' benefits such as free school meals, free prescriptions, mortgage interest and full payment of Housing Benefit, leaving her potentially worse off. If she is receiving Family Credit, the first £15 she receives in maintenance is disregarded and allows her to obtain some extra income. This was intended as a work incentive, but the inducement is meagre compared to potential childcare and other employment costs.

A small-scale in-depth study (Clarke *et al.* 1994) of the early impact of the CSA raised several concerns. No mothers in the study had gained from CSA assessment, and some were worse off. Loss of informal support from fathers – help with clothing, entertainment and presents, etc. – was significant. Enforcing maintenance proved counter-productive – with both parents losing out to the benefit of the taxpayer. Children could suffer financially, and also from a deterioration in relations between parents, and in the quality of contact between parents (especially fathers) and their children.

In July 1999 the government published its plans to reform the system in the White Paper, *A new contract for welfare: Children's Rights and Parents' Responsibilities*. A strong emphasis on parental responsibility remained:

> Every child has the right to the best possible start in life. And parents have a clear responsibility to protect and provide for their

> children so that the children can make the most of their lives. This is a responsibility that endures regardless of family separation.
>
> (DSS 1999, p. 1)

Most changes will take effect in 2001. The basic framework for redistributing resources across households remains, including assessment using a formula and the administrative apparatus of the Child Support Agency. But the formula will be simplified to a flat percentage of the net income of the non-resident parent, based on the number of children and maintaining protection for non-resident parents with low incomes or second families. The government has set lower public expenditure savings targets. Parents with care on Income Support will retain £10 of any child support they receive, before any reduction in their level of benefit and those receiving Working Families Tax Credit will be able to retain all of it.

INTRAHOUSEHOLD RESOURCE TRANSFERS

The Child Support Act affects the level of transfers within 'broken' families, from parents to children. The level of transfers within 'intact' families – intrahousehold transfers – has remained a private concern, with no legal rights guaranteeing individuals a minimum or proportionate share of family resources. Because social security benefits take the household or family as the unit of assessment, they assume that the benefits given to one individual will be distributed equitably to household members, who will share a common standard of living. Do intrahousehold transfers conform to these assumptions?

Research on intrahousehold distribution is difficult, given its 'private' character, the sensitivity of income issues and the potential gulf between principle and practice. Thus it is difficult to distinguish 'personal' income from that contributed to the family coffers. Wilson (1987) argues that mothers tend to feel guilty about using income for personal ends, while fathers often exaggerate their contribution to family resources. Couples may collude in myths about money management bearing little correspondence to how income is actually managed. Producing evidence on resource distribution within families has required intensive qualitative studies, which do not claim to be representative and are hard to replicate.

Pahl's study (1989) of money management among 102 married

couples in Kent in the early 1980s found a high level of commitment to collective views of family income, notably among men who tended to regard it as part of a 'breadwinner' role:

Table 5.4 How do you feel about what you earn? Do you feel it is your income or do you regard it as your husband's/wife's income as well?

Income belongs to	Husband's income		Wife's income	
	His view	Her view	Her view	His view
The earner	7	24	35	52
The couple/family	93	76	65	48
Total	100	100	100	100
Base =	99	100	52	56

Source: Pahl 1984

While both partners tended to regard men's income in collective terms, opinions were more divided over women's income, with men more inclined to regard their wife's income as personal. Most women saw their income as contributing to family resources. In general individuals were more likely to earmark their own income for collective purposes than that of their partners.

Pahl found some disparity between rhetoric and reality, with husbands more inclined to retain personal income in practice, and wives more likely to devote their income to family needs. The extent of income sharing reflected the kind of allocative 'system' the family adopted. Pahl identified several such 'systems':

- **Whole wage system** One partner (usually the wife) is responsible for managing all income and spending.
- **Allowance system** One partner (usually the husband) gives the other an allowance to be spent on specific items, usually for housekeeping, retaining control of remaining income.
- **Pooling system** Both partners have access to all money, and both are responsible for managing it.
- **Independent management system** Both partners have independent income and neither has access to all household funds.

Pahl suggested that women were most vulnerable where the husband kept control of his own earnings and gave his wife an allowance for housekeeping (a quarter of her sample used this system). Men exercised tight control over the budget in about two-thirds of these households.

These issues were also addressed by Vogler (1994) in a study of a large national sample of 1,211 couples using a modified typology of allocative systems. Vogler found that wives were generally more deprived than husbands, an inequality more pronounced under management systems in which wives were primarily responsible for money. Under these systems, inequalities became even greater as income declined, and 'women bore the brunt of both an inadequate total household income and an unequal distribution of income within the home' (Vogler 1994, p. 262). Vogler found:

> The orthodox model of households as egalitarian, decision-making units, within which resources are shared equally, applied to only a fifth of the households in our sample, notably to those using the joint pooling system
>
> (Vogler 1994, p. 241)

A small-scale study (Goode, Callender and Lister 1998) also found gendered patterns of spending, money management and 'going without' by couples on benefit – with women more likely to 'go without', to experience the stress of managing on a low income, and to have less personal spending money. Many women lack access to an adequate income without being dependent on their partners. A study of women at 33 found over half (54%) did not have 'enough to get by' (defined as 140% of Income Support rates) if only their access to independent income was considered (Joshi *et al.* 1995).

Evidence on intrahousehold distribution has implications for policies that aim to reduce poverty, or redistribute resources between households (for example, to those with children). It encourages recognition of rights of individuals within families, and also suggests that ways of paying benefit (notably The Working Families Tax Credit) should not assume an equitable transfer of resources within families.

CONCLUSION

The family redistributes resources among its members, both within households and, in some circumstances, across them. It is important to take account of the distribution of resources that takes place in practice, the inequities that exist in families, and attitudes to meeting obligations to family members. Other resource transfers (gifts for example) may be significant as well as income.

Family policy is redistributive, and support to family incomes can be justified on several (potentially conflicting) grounds. Family policies can redistribute resources vertically from families on higher incomes to those on lower incomes by supplementing income; this is supposed to ensure an adequate minimum standard of living among those on low incomes. Family policies can redistribute resources horizontally to families with children from households without them to achieve greater equity between families. Family policies can also compel a direct redistribution of resources across households, to ensure that private, familial support obligations are fulfilled. However, through inappropriate assumptions, inadequate funding, disincentive effects, and incompetent administration, family policies can be frustrated in many ways.

The Labour government seems committed to both horizontal redistribution and vertical redistribution. Redistributive policies tend to be limited, however, by political constraints – no government likes headlines like those following the 1999 budget: 'Middle class loses out as children gain' (Brown 1999). Different objectives can be difficult to reconcile. Vertical redistribution through more extensive means-testing (such as the WFTC or the new Child Tax Credit) may reduce incentives to work as benefits are withdrawn with rising income. Improving horizontal distribution (for example through increasing Child Benefit) can require high taxation which may bear heavily on those with low incomes. With two budgets in succession hailed as 'budgets for children', the Labour government has attempted (within these constraints) to directly increase the resources reaching families with children, most especially those most in need. But Labour's main approach is to enable families to provide for their own children, by encouraging parents (and especially mothers) to take up paid employment. This use of family policies to alter the balance between home and work is a subject we consider in the next chapter.

KEY POINTS

- Families are economic institutions that transfer, distribute and consume resources. Family policy is redistributive within and between families, vertically from richer to poorer families, and horizontally between families with and without children.
- Greater family and child poverty prompt concern about whether means-tested social security benefits provide an adequate minimum standard of living for families with children. Research shows that families living on social security benefits alone cannot make ends meet.
- Policies can be based on implicit and incorrect assumptions about how families share resources. Most significant for anti-poverty policies is that all family members enjoy a common standard of living. Research shows that resource transfers and management with families show patterns of gender inequality.
- Recent governments have emphasized vertical distribution. Targeting resources on families 'most in need' can create poverty traps. The present government's strategy for families on low incomes is to make paid work economically more rewarding, partly by shifting state support from out-of-work benefits to in-work benefits.
- Equity is important for family policy, since families with children have lower average incomes and greater needs than those without. Child Benefit, a universal benefit to families with children, redistributes income to families with children from those without; but until recently its real value had declined.

GUIDE TO FURTHER READING

For a discussion of adequacy of resources, see:
Berthoud, R. and Ford, R. (1996) 'A new way of measuring relative financial needs' *JRF Findings, Social Policy Research* 109.

For a review of research on standards of living in low-income families, see:
Kempson, E. (1996) *Life on a Low Income,* London: Child Poverty Action Group.

For discussions of equity and child benefit, see:
Bradshaw, J. and Stimson, C. (1997) *Using Child Benefit in the Family Budget,* London: The Stationery Office/SPRU.

Middleton, S., Ashworth, K. and Braithwaite, I. (1997) *Small Fortunes: Spending on children, childhood poverty and parental sacrifice*, York: Joseph Rowntree Foundation.

For details of the distribution of resources within households, see:

Pahl, J. (1989) *Money and Marriage*, London: Macmillan.

Vogler, C. (1994) 'Money in the household' in Anderson, M., Bechhofer, F. and Gershuny, J. (eds) (1994) *The Social and Political Economy of the Household*, Oxford: Oxford University Press.

Goode, J., Callender, C. and Lister, R. (1998) *Purse or Wallet?* London: Policy Studies Institute.

For a review of family incomes policies to the early 1990s, see:

Kamerman, S. B. and Kahn, A. J. (eds) (1997) *Family change and family policies in Great Britain, Canada, New Zealand, and the United States*, Oxford: Clarendon Press, pp. 56–69.

Reconciling work and family life

6

Outline

Paid work is central to New Labour's family policies, for it is seen as enhancing social inclusion and reducing dependency. In this chapter we consider the government's 'family-friendly' employment policies, including policies to increase employment participation (such as childcare provision) and policies to improve the balance between family and employment commitments. We question whether attempts to restructure incentives to work tend to emphasize economic calculation and ignore the influence of family roles on employment decisions. We also ask whether 'family-friendly' policies which do not address more fundamental gender inequalities – in paid and unpaid work – may be either ineffectual or counter-productive. Since time is not elastic, New Labour's emphasis on paid work as a solution to social problems may be hard to reconcile with its professed concern with the needs of family life. It seems that women rather than men will still be expected to square this particular circle.

WORK WITHIN AND OUTSIDE THE FAMILY

> Work offers the surest way for families to provide for themselves. But work also takes up time which could otherwise be committed to the family: caring for children, and also for sick, disabled or elderly family members. Many families find it hard to strike the right balance, and many are suffering from intense pressures on their time. It is in all our interests to reconcile better the demands of work and home.
>
> (Home Office/Ministerial Group on the Family 1998, p. 24)

That families involve work is already evident from the various activities we have considered, such as reproduction, socialization and caring. A distinctive aspect of this work is that it does not involve production for a market – it is not done for pay or profit, and is 'unpaid' labour. Transactions between family members involve exchange, but through reciprocal obligations and commitments that sustain moral reputations and personal worth, rather than cash. Work for the family may meet needs, express personal creativity, or be a means of loving and caring for others. This does not mean that it is 'unproductive' or somehow less onerous, stressful, or challenging than paid employment – despite a bias favouring work for money and devaluing work in the home.

However, any view of 'domestic labour' needs to appreciate the limits of 'reciprocity', given inequalities within families in terms of status, authority and power. Thus work done by children may reflect the authority that parents exercise over them. Because work in the family involves negotiation and maintenance of a moral order, it is free from the formal regulation and control that we associate with employment. Although we speak of a 'division of labour' in the family, it is not the same as the 'division of labour' within the factory or the office. The labour market fills positions through processes of supply and demand, and organizes work through formal specification of time or tasks. Employment is regulated through formal procedures governing aspects of work such as pay, promotion, and performance. It may involve creativity and sociability, but within an instrumental framework oriented to the production of goods and services for sale to others.

From a policy perspective, questions arise about how these different systems – work within and outside the family – intermesh. Each influences an individual's availability and capacity for the other. The labour market cannot operate without a supply of labour, which families provide; and in industrial societies, families cannot realize their aspirations without employment. Here is potential for mutual benefit. On the other hand, both families and labour market require time and commitment, and these may be in short supply. Here is potential for conflict. Paid work offers opportunities but also incurs costs (most obviously, in the time it requires) for family life.

This potential for mutual benefit or conflict has been given added piquancy by the advent of a Labour government committed to both family and work as its core values. The government has acknowledged the need to strike a balance between time for each, since time is not elastic. It has also identified work as 'the surest way for families to provide for themselves', and pursued policies aimed at maximizing employment. Although this tension may, in the short-run, prove productive, it may ultimately prove destructive and self-defeating.

'FAMILY-FRIENDLY' POLICIES

The 'breadwinner' model does not describe our image of most families today. We no longer assume a sharp division between men inhabiting the public domain of paid work, and women inhabiting the private domain of homemaking and childcare or informal care. Compared with the breadwinner model of one parent working and one at home, more families now have either two earners, or no earners at all, producing a growing disparity between 'work rich' and 'work poor' families. For those with two earners, family life now involves a juggling act between home and work, often resulting in a dual burden for women, and the stresses of having either too much or too little work. Family policies have been concerned with helping mothers in particular to combine work within and outside the family.

British policies to support parents have been described as 'conservative and hesitant' compared to those of our European counterparts (Kamerman and Kahn 1997, p. 47). In the 1980s and 1990s, the lead for family-friendly employment policies came from the European Union. The typical story was of an EU directive that the UK government resisted – obstructing it altogether, weakening its provisions, or conceding grudgingly to its obligations under EU law. British resistance to the EU legislation to limit working time to a weekly average of 48 hours was indicative of political indifference to the conflicting demands of work in the family and employment. However, this stance may be changing, as the Labour government introduces 'family-friendly' employment policies as one part of its programme 'to rebuild the welfare state around work'. Family-friendly policies are conceived as work-friendly policies, although the centrality of work is related to other considerations, such as reducing welfare bills. But can the objectives of raising employment participation and achieving a better balance between employment and family life be reconciled?

WOMEN'S INCREASING PARTICIPATION IN EMPLOYMENT

A striking feature of changes in labour supply during the 1980s and 1990s was the convergence of men's and women's participation in the labour market. The economic activity rate for women aged 16–59 rose from 62% in 1975 to 73% in 1995; over the same period, the economic activity of men aged 16–64 fell from 93% to 86% (ONS 1997 Tables 4.1 and 4.2). The fall in male activity was far greater among older workers; by 1995 a fifth of men over 50 and a half of those aged 60–64 were no longer economically active (ONS 1997 Table 4.3). But fathers with dependent children are more likely than other men to be in paid work, and most employed fathers (over 90%) work full-time.

The rise in female economic activity rates was entirely due to an increase in the number of married women in employment – the rates for non-married women actually fell slightly (ONS 1997 Table 4.2). One contributing factor has been the increasing proportion of women with dependent children in paid employment, which by 1995, had risen to almost two-thirds (Table 6.1). Other evidence shows that increases were the greatest among mothers with children under 5, for whom participation rates doubled (27% to 55%) in the same period.

Table 6.1 Economic activity of women of working age (16–59) with dependent children, 1973–1995 Great Britain

	1973	1995
All economically active	49	66
Unemployed	2	6
All working	47	60
Working full-time	17	22
Working part-time	30	38
Base = 100%	4,441	2,944

Source: Derived from ONS 1997 Table 4.7

These trends have changed the policy agenda. The absence of 'working mothers' from the family provokes anxiety among those who believe her proper place is in the home. This view still enjoys considerable currency, apparent in the media's delight over the failure of some women executives to 'make it' in a 'man's world'. As this emphasis on a maternal role is hard to reconcile with demand for female employees, the policies of the Conservative administrations were ambivalent and – whenever labour seemed in short supply – contradictory. The Labour government has tried to square the circle by focusing on the central role of work in 'providing' for families, reducing emphasis on parental time with children. Hence the key role of childcare provision in Labour's programme.

However, current policies also address three problems which have become pressing with the rise in female employment:

- the prevalence of part-time work and its implications for low pay and unequal opportunity
- a growing division between 'work rich' and work poor' families
- the failure of lone mothers to share in the general rise in female employment.

Let's briefly consider each in turn.

The sharpest rises in female participation have been in part-time employment, although more women with dependent children were also working full-time. Women are still expected to adjust their labour market activities to accommodate their domestic responsibilities. Patterns of adjustment reflect the number of children; the fewer the children, the more likely mothers are to work and to work full-time (Table 6.2).

Table 6.2 Women of working age (16–59) with dependent children working full-time or part-time, 1995 Great Britain

	Full-time %	Part-time %
Number of dependent children		
One	29	37
Two	20	42
Three or more	12	32
All with dependent children	22	38

Source: Derived from ONS 1997 Table 4.8

Part-time work may be a positive way of adjusting to the demands of home and work. But women working part-time tend to have low-skilled, low-paid jobs with poor conditions and promotion prospects. This may waste skilled labour, notably through occupational downgrading on return to part-time work after childbirth (McRae 1991; Callender 1996). It may also reduce financial independence and increase claims for state subsidies such as Family Credit or the Working Families Tax Credit.

Families are increasingly 'work rich' or 'work poor'; both two-earner and no-earner families have become more common. Between 1971 and 1991, the proportion of households of working-age couples in which no one worked rose from 3% to 9%, while the proportion of two-earner couples rose from 46% to 60%. In 1997, more than half (52%) of couples with a pre-school-age child both worked; rising to nearly three-quarters (74%) for couples whose youngest child was 10 or older (Burghes, Clarke and Cronin 1997, p. 46).

The increase in two-earner families attests to the demise of the 'male breadwinner' model of the family. Men remain the main earners for most couples, but women's earnings are an increasingly significant component of family income that protects many families from poverty. Using data from the General Household Survey from 1979–1991, Harkness, Machin and Waldfogel (1994) found that women working part-time contributed 20% to family income on average, while women working full-time contributed over 40%. For couples with children, women's earnings contribution rose by 50%, while the share of family income from men's earnings fell, especially from low-paid men. Women's earnings moderated the rise in poverty and inequalities between families, underlining the problems of families altogether excluded from the labour.

Among these families, we can increasingly include those headed by lone mothers, whose employment levels actually fell over the two decades to 1995 (Table 6.3).

Table 6.3 Married women and lone mothers with dependent children working full-time or part-time, 1977–1995 Great Britain

	1977–1979 %		1993–1995 %	
Married women working	52		65	
Working full-time		15		23
Working part-time		37		42
Lone mothers working	47		40	
Working full-time		22		16
Working part-time		24		24

Source: Derived from ONS 1997 Table 4.10

The Labour government has responded to these trends with a range of measures, including some – notably benefit cuts and conditions – with a rather punitive aspect. The main carrot combined with this stick has been the National Childcare Strategy, to improve provision of accessible, affordable, high quality childcare.

CHILDCARE POLICIES

Childcare by adults other than parents can meet several objectives. It can benefit a child's development and education. It can benefit parents by enabling them to participate in employment. It can benefit employers and society by enlarging and improving the labour supply. Childcare provision can be considered an investment, particularly if it reduces benefit claims and expands tax revenues by increasing employment. Ward *et al.* (1996), reviewing the experience of 33-year-old mothers in the National Child Development Survey, argue that lack of formal full-time childcare may limit women's opportunities to achieve short- and long-term financial independence, particularly if they work part-time in low-paid employment and are obliged to rely on informal family support. Differential access to childcare may reinforce a growing polarity between those earning high salaries and those who are not.

Childcare takes many forms, including nurseries, nannies, workplace crèches, playgroups, registered childminders and after-school and vacation care, plus informal childcare by family, friends and neighbours. Policy debates on childcare have centred on pre-school provision. Public pre-school childcare provision has been traditionally divided between education services, providing pre-school education, and social services, providing daycare for the children of working parents.

Childcare provision

Britain approached the millennium with some of the poorest public childcare provision in the EU. Many working mothers organize work commitments so that childcare is not needed. The DfEE Family and Working Lives Survey 1996–1997 survey found that 40% of working mothers of pre-school children reported that other carers were not needed because they only worked during school hours, worked at home or took their children to work with them. Those needing childcare were particularly dependent on informal support (Table 6.4). Fewer than one in ten were able to depend only on formal provision, leaving them at the mercy of prevailing moralities, whatever their own inclinations or the financial consequences for the family.

Table 6.4 Packages of childcare used by employed mothers
Working-age wives with dependent children Great Britain

	Married mothers %	Lone mothers %
Percentage who used:		
Formal/school	3	2
Informal/formal/school	2	3
Other package	3	3
Other care	4	5
No usual care arrangement	4	4
Informal/formal	5	4
Formal care	9	6
School	12	17
Informal/school	16	22
Informal care	40	35

Source: Ward, Dale and Joshi (1996 Table 1)

With two-thirds of children living in households where both parents work, lack of good quality, accessible and affordable childcare remains an issue despite the expansion of formal childcare provision in the 1990s. Users of formal childcare are more likely to be in full-time work with higher incomes and higher status occupations, in dual-earner households. Lone parents face the greatest obstacles in obtaining affordable care, which is a major barrier to seeking employment. Some simple sums suggest the level of childcare provision is too low. There are 830,000 registered childcare places compared to 5.1 million children aged under 8 in England (DfEE and DSS 1998). Of children aged 3–5, 60% have some form of public nursery care, but this figure drops to less than 5% for the under 3s (Family Policy Studies Centre 1998b, p. 7).

One established approach to supporting families with childcare has been to subsidize parents rather than fund public provision. Parents on Family Credit have been eligible for a childcare disregard for formal rather than informal childcare costs since 1994, i.e. income used to pay for formal childcare is disregarded when calculating entitlement to Family Credit. Vouchers to pay for public and private pre-school care and tax allowances for formal childcare costs have been considered but not generally adopted as policy options.

Cohen and Fraser (1991) emphasize the role of the public sector in stimulating or providing services, outlining 'principles' upon which policy should be based:

- Provision must be equitable and responsive.
- Childcare must encompass education and care.
- Policies on childcare and employment must be linked.

In 1998, the government published a consultation document with its National Childcare Strategy (DfEE and DSS 1998, Cm 3959). The main proposals, some already implemented, were to:

- create 50,000 pre-school childcare places in 1998/1999
- double the number of out-of-school places for school-age children
- provide universal non-compulsory nursery education for all 4 year olds
- double the number of nursery places for 3 year olds
- establish Early Excellence Centres to disseminate good practice
- set up a helpline for parents to find out what is available
- raise Child Benefit to improve affordability of childcare
- introduce a new childcare tax credit, as part of the new Working Families Tax Credit
- improve the quality of childcare by a more stringent system of regulation and training of childcarers.

This policy represents a clear shift from the previous market-based approach to more public and institutional forms of childcare. But concerns remain. These include the cost and supply of childcare places for the under 3s; whether childcare places on the scale and of the quality required will materialize; whether pre-school care will be flexible and affordable enough; and whether the policy leaves parents who prefer to look after their own children with enough support (Family Policy Studies Centre 1998b).

Childcare, economics and employment

Deeper issues are raised by family policies aimed at improving childcare provision. Accounts of labour market activity usually focus on individual economic calculation to explain behaviour. This is apparent in debates about employment among lone parents. Those embracing the 'underclass' thesis have argued that welfare benefits are too high, encouraging lone parents to live on benefit. Others have argued that lack of affordable childcare is a major constraint preventing lone mothers (and others) from taking up employment. Both perspectives tend to assume a rational calculation of costs and benefits of working on the part of (lone) mothers. They tend to 'construct' poor people as rational egotistical opportunists out to exploit opportunities provided by the welfare system, or as passive victims systematically victimized and marginalized by public policies.

Evidence suggests that policies based upon abstract models of economic calculation may bear very little relation to the social realities which families experience. A study of claimants leaving Family Credit found low-income families had a poor level of knowledge about their eligibility for means-tested benefits – even where they have had recent experience of claiming it (Bryson and Marsh 1996, pp. 71–72). Family Credit 'had only marginal significance' in decisions about employment when compared with other factors families took into account, most notably good wages, security and reliable childcare (Bryson and Marsh 1996, pp. 77–78). A 1993 survey of 9,000 lone parents in receipt of Family Credit found that only 5% saw it as the major incentive to work. Reliable childcare, good wages and security were ranked as 'most important' – in that order. Whether the Working Families Tax Credit will change matters remains to be seen.

Economic and social decisions

Edwards and Duncan (1996) argue that the orthodox approach offers an unconvincing (and inconsistent) account of labour market behaviour. People do not act like rational economic calculating machines. They act in a social context, influenced by social moralities and identities, particularly in a family setting. Of course economists do sometimes recognize the existence of families, but the economic approach tends to treat the family as an economic nexus in which the household allocates labour to maximize resources – as if it were a mini-labour market. Or they tend to treat the family as irrelevant because it is basically about social relationships not economic activity. However, it is misleading to see the family as a place where people make social decisions but not economic ones; and equally misleading to see the labour market as an arena where people make economic decisions and not social ones.

People may be influenced by costs and benefits, but they are also influenced by other considerations, like what is involved in being a good mum. It makes a difference if women are regarded (and regard themselves) predominantly as mothers or as workers – and this can vary from place to place and time to time. Edwards and Duncan suggest that social moralities operate at a local level, explaining wide variations in employment rates among lone mothers in different localities. Local labour markets have an effect, but this is mediated (they suggest) by how women are integrated into employment. High levels of employment among lone mothers are found where local traditions of women working full-time are strong, and vice versa. Local traditions may affect both expectations and levels of practical support. They may also affect the recruitment expectations (and location decisions) of employers. Hence mothers may end up in part-time jobs – or not in employment at all.

Variations in employment rates reflect national as well as local 'social moralities'. Compare the 40% of lone mothers in paid employment in Britain (16% full-time) – with 58% in Germany (35% full-time); and 87% in Sweden (33% full-time). International comparisons are complicated – many of Sweden's part-timers work longer hours than Britain's full-timers. But these variations are very striking. In Germany breadwinners (including lone mothers) can earn a 'family wage', supported also by the tax system, because mothers generally are expected to stay at home. In Sweden all parents (including lone mothers) are expected to work, so account is taken of their needs through extensive childcare provision and reduced hours of work. In Britain we neither assume one thing nor the other. We do not assume mothers will work – so there is little formal childcare provision. We do not assume mothers will not work – so there is little support for a family wage. This may give lone mothers choice – or the worst of all worlds, where lack of childcare and low wages combine to make it difficult for lone mothers to work.

The limitations of 'rational economic man'

Some support for these arguments can be found in an earlier neighbourhood study of the labour market decisions of a small number of families (36) in a white working class estate in Exeter (Jordan *et al.* 1992). This too stressed the limitations of 'rational economic man' and importance of how people construct identities and roles in a social context. The researchers assumed that people actively shape their lives and make choices about things like labour market activity or living off benefits, in ways which reflect the roles they take on as husbands and wives. In this account people are neither pathologically depraved nor passive victims – but active, resourceful and above all concerned to construct themselves as 'morally' adequate in terms of family responsibilities.

The men on this estate embraced a dual role – as 'worker' and 'provider'. As workers, men stressed the challenging nature of work that contributed to one's sense of moral worth. As providers, they emphasized their role in supporting the family financially – with earnings seen as a 'family wage' even if insufficient. These roles could be hard to reconcile. Most men had irregular work patterns, often working while on benefit without declaring their earnings. As 'workers' this was legitimated in terms of keeping active, since idleness undermined identity and self-respect. As 'providers', it was legitimated in terms of responsibility to provide an adequate family income. That did not mean that men were reconciled to living off benefit. Most would take a regular job consistent with their sense of moral adequacy as workers and providers. Most would work overtime despite the disincentive effects of losing extra income through taxes and lost benefits. As the researchers comment:

> it is their construction of their identities as workers and providers which causes men to be relatively impervious to these disincentive effects on taking employment or increasing earnings
>
> (Jordan *et al.* 1992, p. 130)

Women were also aware of disincentive effects, preferring not to do 'one night for the taxman'. They also responded to the disincentive effects of losing benefit income if earning while their partners were unemployed. But the major influence on their labour market behaviour was their role as mothers:

> The preponderance of part-time work among our women respondents is constructed by the women themselves as taking this form because of their children's needs
>
> (Jordan *et al.* 1992, p. 158)

Their first priority was to meet their children's needs through care, with income and personal fulfilment as secondary considerations. Women were also affected by their husband's role: his willingness (or otherwise) to help at home was 'a very important determinant of women's labour supply decisions' (Jordan *et al.* 1992, p. 170). If their partner did not help, women relied on friends or relatives, especially to care for younger children, for whom more formal childcare was rejected as inappropriate.

Both partners struggled to sustain credible family roles in circumstances that conspired to undermine them. Men had difficulty in acting as 'providers', while women had problems reconciling their maternal roles with the availability of regular employment and the vital contribution their income could make to family finances.

Such studies suggest in different ways that decisions about employment are much more complex than allowed by simple economic models. Policies that shift the balance of economic calculation – for example, by subsidizing childcare – may be frustrated by other factors, more intangible perhaps but also more intransigent, such as prevailing perceptions of parental roles and responsibilities.

WORK-TIME POLICIES

Family-friendly policies include ways of altering work-time to allow adults to reconcile family and work commitments more readily.

> The vast majority of people raise children at some point in their working lives, and have to adjust their lives to cope. A significant proportion – about one in four – also have responsibilities as carers for elderly, sick or disabled people. Many people want to be able to provide care within the family or to look after their children, while also benefiting from greater independence through paid employment. They often need part time work or work with flexible hours. For all of these people flexible family-friendly working arrangements are essential for helping them to balance their family responsibilities with paid employment. The availability of childcare, flexible working arrangements and reasonable time off to deal with family emergencies, all contribute to making it possible for everyone to share in the social and economic benefits of work
>
> (Home Office/Ministerial Group on the Family 1998, p. 24)

Although considered mainly in terms of the needs of parents, 'family-friendly' policies may also accommodate the needs of carers to adjust their working hours to meet the more unpredictable demands for care from sick children or infirm relatives. These demands are usually unpredictable in frequency and duration (Brannen *et al.* 1994). In the absence of flexible employment arrangements they make it difficult for carers to combine their responsibilities with (full-time) employment.

Family-friendly policies can include:

- maternity rights and benefits
- maternity and paternity leave
- parental and family leave
- regular reduced working hours
- arrangements for emergency leave
- provision for working from home
- flexitime
- career breaks
- job sharing
- work during school hours or term-time only
- annual hours contracts.

In general, other European countries have been leading the way:

- In all European countries women are entitled to leave after childbirth. Four EU countries provide statutory paternity leave and twelve provide statutory parental leave, ranging from 3 months for each parent (Greece) to 3 years in total (Germany).
- In Denmark public sector and almost all private sector employees are entitled to paid leave on the first day of a child's illness. In France all women in the public sector can take 12 days leave a year to look after a sick child. In Ireland civil servants can take 5 days paid leave for this purpose.
- Sweden was the first EU country to introduce parental leave for fathers (in 1974). Nearly half of fathers take leave, averaging 43 days, during their child's first year. Almost all mothers (98%) take leave, averaging 262 days, so gender differences remain, although better-educated parents are more likely to share childcare responsibilities (Hantrais and Letablier 1996, p. 127).

In Britain, working hours have been increasing rather than decreasing. Men's working hours are now among the longest in

Europe. In 1995 men worked 45 hours per week on average; 40% worked 46 hours or more per week. Fathers especially work long hours. In 1993, fathers of children under 11 in full-time work averaged 48 hours per week; a high proportion worked over 50 hours. Fathers of very young children in one-earner families work even longer hours: averaging 55 hours per week (Burghes, Clarke and Cronin 1997, p. 44). Such long hours may seriously inhibit a father's ability to share in domestic work. Reviewing the evidence, Utting (1995) suggests that long hours have a damaging impact on the quality of family life.

Increasing female participation

Employers (especially in the public sector) have responded to rising female participation, with over three-quarters making some provision for women with children, such as time off for emergencies or flexible, non-standard hours. But few employers (about one in ten) offer practical help with children and even fewer (about one in 50) operate a workplace crèche or nursery. The 'granny crèche' established by Coventry employers to assist employees caring for elderly infirm relatives remains the exception rather than the rule.

'Flexible' work has become more common, reported by 10% of men and 15% of women. However, it is difficult to judge whether and how far these more flexible forms of working benefit parents, as much depends on whether flexible hours are adjusted to meet their needs or those of their employers. Work during unsocial hours (evenings, nights or weekends) is increasing for men in both single- and dual-earner families. They may make joint family activities less likely, with consequences for the quality of family life (Burghes, Clarke and Cronin 1997, p. 45).

Nor may women benefit as much as one might expect from greater flexibility in the labour market. A study of nursing cited by Cooper (1998) attributed female disadvantage (male nurses climb the career ladder much more quickly, despite women having better qualifications and more experience) to family-friendly arrangements such as career breaks and part-time work patterns. As debates in Sweden suggests, family-friendly policies oriented to or taken up mainly by women may sideline rather than advance their labour market careers. Part-time work has become an important means by which women meet the dual demands of paid work and family, but often at an unreasonable cost in terms of levels of remuneration and conditions of work. Although part-time work is making in-roads into managerial and professional occupations, particularly in the public sector, it more often acts as a trap confining women returning to the labour market to low-paid, low-status jobs with few prospects of promotion. Hence the importance of arrangements allowing women to return to the labour market after childbirth on a full-time basis.

Maternity rights were introduced in 1975, and amended several times in the 1980s, making them more complex and less generous in scope and eligibility. Eligibility depends on meeting criteria such as a minimum period of continuous employment with the same employer and working for a minimum number of hours. Maternity pay was introduced in 1978 for some workers and was replaced in 1987 by Statutory Maternity Pay, whose amount is linked to a worker's length of service. Many women workers were excluded from these benefits because their employment history did not meet the qualifying criteria (Gauthier 1996, p. 173). The EU Pregnant Workers Directive in 1994 forced Britain to change. Paid maternity leave for a minimum of 14 weeks was introduced at least at the level of statutory sick pay, with no minimum length of service required. At present, if the qualifying criteria are met, the benefits include statutory maternity pay, paid time off for antenatal care, employment protection against dismissal because of pregnancy, and a right to return to work (to a similar, but not necessarily the same, job) after a postnatal period (Kamerman and Kahn 1997, p. 51). The 1999 Budget has reduced the qualification conditions so that from August 2000 all mothers-to-be in work earning £30 a week or more (about 95% of all women in work) will qualify for 18 weeks maternity pay.

Parental leave

In contrast to maternity leave around the time of a birth, there is as yet (at the time of writing) no statutory provision for parental leave or family leave (paid or unpaid). The previous government's non-interventionist stance on employer/employee relations viewed such matters as best negotiated privately between them. Flexible working arrangements, reduced hours to meet family commitments, and access to childcare were *ad hoc* and patchy on the whole, with no statutory entitlements or provision. The present government (DTI 1998) proposes a number of 'family-friendly' employment policies as part of its welfare to work strategy. These include implementing several EU directives:

- The EU Parental Leave Directive (by 1999) gives parents the right to 3 months' unpaid leave after the birth or adoption of a child and time off for urgent family reasons, with the guarantee of their own, or a comparable, job on their return.
- Maternity leave is extended to 18 weeks, to match the period of maternity pay. There is to be a review of the whole package of maternity rights and benefits.
- The EU Part-Time Work Directive removes (by 2000) discrimination against part-time workers' entitlements to employment rights.
- The EU Working Time Directive limits the working week to 48 hours unless employees themselves want to work longer.

While these are steps in the right direction, they may have only a marginal impact on working patterns and their impact may be limited by weak implementation. The introduction of the 48-hour week, for example, may be so hedged around with caveats as to have little real impact on working hours (Hewitt 1993). The 48 Hour Working Time Directive is flexibly framed (it allows an average of 48 hours over 17 weeks) and allows for many exemptions. Even so the Labour government has weakened its impact still further by allowing those in professional occupations to please themselves with regard to 'voluntary' working hours. It is unlikely that the Directive will have much impact on British working hours (currently the longest in Europe), although decisions allowing claims by individual employees over long hours and stress-related illness may give the legislation more bite. The introduction of limited rights to parental leave and extension of maternity pay may encourage the trend for mothers to return to full-time work but will have little impact on the gendered patterns of combining employment and child-rearing.

Work-time policies may even in some respects prove ineffectual or even counter-productive. Improvements in the status and conditions of part-time work may reduce its availability. If women can more easily combine work and family commitments, this may reduce the pressure for change in male work patterns.

Changing gender roles

Harker (1996, p. 48) suggests that family-friendly policies should:

- enable people to fulfil family as well as work demands
- promote gender equality and the sharing of family responsibilities

- be non-discriminatory, employee-friendly and accompanied by acceptable working conditions
- strike a balance between the needs of employees and employer.

Increased participation of men in family life is likely to prove the most elusive of these objectives. To appreciate the problems involved in changing gender roles, we must consider how work is organized in the home.

One review of research on the relationship between families and employment drew the conclusion that the evidence suggests that men are more involved in domestic work, particularly those with employed partners who work full-time – but they still do much less housework and childcare than women (Brannen *et al.* 1994). In short, 'We have many "new women" but they are suffering from a dearth of "new men"' (Willetts 1993, p. 8).

A later study is more optimistic, finding that fathers are spending more time with their children and becoming more emotionally involved with them (Burghes, Clarke and Cronin 1997). In this study 45% of mothers and 50% of fathers claimed that childcare was shared equally. Other studies (reviewed in Burghes, Clarke and Cronin 1997, pp. 60–63) suggest that behaviour has been slower to change. Although men do more than before, women still do the great bulk of domestic work. The Office for National Statistics (1998) reported that eight out of ten women still did the domestic chores and only 1% of men did washing, ironing or decided what to have for dinner. Even where women work full-time, they remain the partner with primary responsibility for housework.

One reason this may be so can be discerned in a study (Dench 1996) exploring views of men's role in the family. Dench interviewed 221 respondents, in East London, about half from ethnic communities. About half his respondents were 'traditional' in outlook, seeing the family as a network of rights and obligations based on marriage and a conventional division of labour. About one-third embraced an 'alternative' perspective, seeing the family as a private concern, defined as partners saw fit, with personal autonomy as a fundamental value. Most advocating alternative views saw a role for men in the family as important – but also optional and subject to negotiation. Dench observes that this could lead to men reducing their commitment to family work, suggesting that departures from the 'traditional' division of labour may not always involve a greater participation by men in family life.

Innovative work patterns within families were examined in a study of Australian families, based on in-depth interviews with 50 couples in Sidney who did things 'differently' (Goodnow and Bowes 1994, p. 3, p. 37) – the main difference being that one person accepted responsibility for a 'non-conventional' area of work. Work divisions were based on various criteria, including:

- availability for the job
- competence for the job
- each person's likes and dislikes
- the standards to which the work should be done.

Respect for likes and dislikes and for different standards proved major factors shaping work patterns. Couples negotiated within a moral framework in which work 'is a way by which people signal what they think of themselves, what they expect of others, how they feel about others, and what they regard as fair or just' (Goodnow and Bowes 1994, p. 2). They were concerned above all to respect the values and choices of their partners – for example, avoiding the unfairness of allowing one partner to get stuck with all the jobs that both dislike. In general, distinctions based on gender had been displaced by concerns about 'sharing, choice, efficiency or the simple justice of both people contributing' (Goodnow and Bowes 1994, p. 182).

Couples not only allocate unpaid work within the home; they also make decisions about paid work outside of the home; and each of these decisions is likely to influence the other. How do families reconcile (if at all) the competing demands for care and career? Recent research has tried to understand parents as situated social actors and how couples come to make investments in particular combinations of domestic work and employment. The way people make such investments can be explained partly in terms of long-term strategic bargaining (Jordan *et al.* 1994, p. 150). In allocating scarce resources (time) people may take account of both short-term and long-term returns. In doing so, they have to take their partner's strategies into account. Economic calculation does not suffice, for couples have to sustain trust and commitment over time in order to realize their personal investments, especially where investments are 'asymmetric' with men investing more heavily in careers and women more heavily in the home. Therefore bargaining requires a moral framework, in which partners facilitate personal autonomy through 'the exchange of ritual respect in partnership' (Jordan *et al.* 1994, p. 151). Bargaining on the basis of such a 'partnership code' is rarely explicit – couples can seldom articulate a rational account of decisions. The 'partnership code' is less a set of moral principles regulating behaviour than a stock of cultural resources allowing partners to interpret behaviour in divergent ways, and giving scope for flexibility in adapting to changing circumstances. It provides a way of regulating conflicts, in relationships characterized by 'asymmetric power relations', as both partners have 'enough autonomy to pursue their own purposes and interests within the relationship' (Jordan *et al.* 1994, p. 174).

Why do many women invest so heavily in the home and so little in their own employment assets? Jordan and colleagues suggest that in a partnership context, women make personal short-term sacrifices and accept medium-term risks to achieve long-term gains. This brings an immediate return, if a highly segmented labour market offers far higher returns to men than to women. By supporting their partner's career, women may obtain a longer-term return in terms of their partner's higher pension after retirement. However, once women opt for a supportive role, they may find 'that it is too late to go back and be forced to start from a very disadvantaged position' in developing their own job assets (Jordan *et al.* 1994, p. 157). Given that four in ten marriages may end in divorce, such strategies clearly involve substantial risks for women.

CONCLUSION

These studies, in their different ways, underline the importance of moral and cultural as well as economic forces in shaping changes in the domestic division of labour and the prospects for improving the participation of men in family life. They suggest that underlying structural factors – such as gender inequalities in the labour market itself – may have an important influence on the strategies which people pursue in balancing their commitments to family and employment.

For these reasons, the goals of 'family-friendly' policies may prove elusive, especially if they produce only marginal changes in labour market expectations. Paradoxically, policies which on paper offer opportunities to achieve a better balance between family and work may in practice reinforce traditional divisions. This is not to suggest that policies to improve childcare or make work-time more flexible are misconceived. Policies themselves can contribute to significant change in the climate of opinion. But it does suggest that the challenge of changing current work/family patterns, and particularly the gender imbalance, will require a vigorous, thorough and comprehensive approach, not only to extending employment opportunities for women, but also to improving the incentives for men to care. Whether a Labour government that sees 'work' as the route to salvation can embrace both of these goals with equal determination remains to be seen.

KEY POINTS

- The 'breadwinner' model of the family is increasingly replaced by either two earners juggling the dual burden of home and work – or no earners. Men work less and married women more, especially part-time, although men remain the main earners for most families. Women's earnings are a significant component of family income that provides protection from poverty. Fathers' working hours, working unsocial hours and 'flexible' work have all increased, making joint family activities more difficult, and potentially damaging the quality of family life.
- Women's greater participation in paid work is not matched by men's increased participation in family life. Although attitudes to gender roles in the family are more egalitarian, and men work more at home than in the past, men's behaviour has been slower to change than women's.
- Work within and outside the family influence each other and have the potential for mutual benefit or conflict. Research shows that couples' decisions about paid employment involve more than simple economic calculations, they also involve social and moral decisions such as children's need for care by their parents.
- Family-friendly policies include ways of altering work-time to allow adults to reconcile family and work commitments more readily, such as maternity rights and benefits, various forms of leave from work for parents and carers, and reduced and more flexible working time. So far British policies to support working parents have been 'conservative and hesitant' compared to other European countries.

- Recent childcare policies, shifting from earlier market-based approaches, aim to expand Britain's public and institutional childcare provision, which are currently among the poorest in the EU. Lack of good quality, accessible and affordable childcare remains a major work disincentive.

GUIDE TO FURTHER READING

For more about the UK and EC 'family-friendly' employment policies, see:

Kamerman, S. B. and Kahn, A. J. (eds) (1997) *Family change and family policies in Great Britain, Canada, New Zealand, and the United States*, Oxford: Clarendon Press, pp. 47– 55.

Hantrais, L. and Letablier, M. (1996) *Families and Family Policies in Europe*, London: Longman.

For a brief review of UK childcare policies since the Second World War, see:

Kamerman, S. B. and Kahn, A. J. (eds) (1997) *Family change and family policies in Great Britain, Canada, New Zealand, and the United States*, Oxford: Clarendon Press, pp. 70–79.

For a review of research on men's and women's domestic division of labour, see:

Burghes, L., Clarke, L. and Cronin, N. (1997) *Fathers and fatherhood in Britain*, London: Family Policy Studies Centre.

A new family policy? 7

Outline
Although family policy in Britain is conventionally regarded as implicit rather than explicit, New Labour have placed the family (along with work) at the centre of their social policy agenda. In this chapter, we trace the evolution of family policy over the years, setting New Labour's approach in the context of the post-war and Thatcher periods. We suggest that New Labour's attempt to develop a 'third way' between traditional and libertarian perspectives is rooted in the party's traditions as well as evidence of the impact of New Right thinking on the importance of responsibilities as well as rights. New Labour is also changing the institutional framework within which family policies are developed, but we express some doubts as to whether this represents a fundamental break with the traditional British approach to family policy.

STATE INTERVENTION IN THE FAMILY

> A modern family policy needs to recognise these new realities [of family life] ... First the interests of children must be paramount. The Government's interest in family policy is primarily an interest in ensuring that the next generation gets the best possible start in life.
> (Home Office/Ministerial Group on the Family 1998, p. 4)

Britain generally has pursued a broadly non-interventionist approach, with selective intervention based on need. But in 1997, the Labour government established a Ministerial Group on the Family, headed by the Home Secretary. It has pursued 'joined up' policies on the family through the Supporting Families Green Paper (Home Office/Ministerial Group on the Family 1998), Labour's two budgets (both hailed – or 'hyped' – as budgets for children and families) and other initiatives including the National Carers Strategy, the National Childcare Strategy and the family-friendly policies of *The Fairness at Work* White Paper.

The government claims its family policy is pragmatic, neither traditional nor libertarian:

> Just as the strains on families have increased over the years, so the support provided to help families needs to change too. Neither a 'back to basics' fundamentalism, trying to turn back the clock, nor an 'anything goes' liberalism which denies the fact that how families behave affects us all, is credible any more.
> (Home Office/Ministerial Group on the Family 1998, p. 5)

Is Britain developing an explicit family policy, where the state adopts a more substantial and overt role in supporting families? As the Labour government is in its infancy, any answer must be tentative. But we can at least consider Labour's claims to be making a break with the past by reviewing how family policy developed over the post-war era. We can divide this whistle-stop tour into three main periods: the post-war consensus, the Conservative era from 1979 and the Labour period from 1997. In reviewing family policies over this period, we must attend to both family policy *outputs*, i.e. 'specific measures, legislation and orientation, which characterized a government's support for families' and family policy *inputs*, i.e. 'factors which may have influenced the policy-making process and the adoption of specific policies' (Gauthier 1996, p. 3, p. 4).

THE POST-WAR CONSENSUS: 1945–1979

The British approach in the earlier part of the twentieth century assumed that the state should not promote policies for all families but only play a marginal role where serious problems existed in 'problem families'. During the inter-war period, some attention was given to mothers and children in low-income families, stimulated by Eleanor Rathbone's campaign for family allowances. The Second World War gave the political impetus for a change in direction for family policy. The Beveridge Report (1942) called for replacement of the 'poor law' framework by a limited universalism in social security provisions for all families.

The Beveridge Report

Despite its reforming rhetoric, the Beveridge Report was more modest in the detail of its ambitions, focusing on an integrated system of national insurance and a safety net of national social assistance. While these were significant achievements, adoption of flat-rate benefits at or below subsistence levels stored up future trouble. So too did a presumption that insurance was mainly to provide for male breadwinners suffering temporary interruptions in employment. So structured, the insurance system could not cope with high levels of long-term unemployment, leading to an increasingly heavy dependence on means-tested assistance. The system was ill-adapted to changes in family structure as well as employment, likewise resulting in a shift to means-tested benefits as a method of family support.

The Beveridge Report made important assumptions about family structure and responsibility which have shaped our social security system and wider welfare provision. For example, the Report states:

> In any measure of social policy in which regard is had to facts, the great majority of married women must be regarded as occupied on work which is vital though unpaid, without which their husbands could not do their paid work and without which the nation could not continue. In accord with facts the Plan for Social Security treats married women as a special insurance class of occupied persons and treats man and wife as a team.
>
> (Beveridge 1942, p. 49)

> She [the married woman] has other duties ... The Plan ... puts a premium on marriage in place of penalising it. ... In the next thirty years housewives as mothers have vital work to do in ensuring the adequate continuance of the British Race and British Ideals in the World.
>
> (Beveridge 1942, p. 52)

Families were assumed to conform to a 'breadwinner' model in which women's primary role is in the home while men act as breadwinners. Marriages were assumed to be enduring and provide life-long support. Beveridge endorsed an orthodoxy as yet undisturbed (despite women's war-time role) by post-war social and economic change. However, this left the social security system ill-adapted to cope with what was to come.

The reforms focused on the state, and made no explicit provision for all families – with the partial exception of family allowances, introduced in 1945 for families with two or more children, and extended to cover the first child in 1975. The family was seen as a private domain where non-intervention was desirable. Families could call on the new provisions for education and health services, and more selectively, social housing, to support their welfare activities. But welfare provisions favoured some families over others.

The 1960s and 1970s

This was the framework through which family policies were formed in the post-war period. The 'rediscovery of poverty' in the 1960s put family poverty back on the political agenda. The poverty lobby emerged, including the pressure groups Child Poverty Action Group in 1965 and Shelter in 1966. Policies in social security, health and family law became more explicit in their efforts to support families and also began to recognize their changing character. Notable in this respect were reform of family allowances, abortion policies, and divorce law reform. Family poverty – notably the Labour government's failure to reduce it – became an issue in the 1970 election.

In the 1970s concern with poor families rose with unemployment. Redistributive policies were introduced to benefit families in poverty. Family Income Supplement, a means-tested benefit for low-income families in full-time work was introduced in 1971. The Finer Committee on One Parent Families reported in 1974, recommending a guaranteed maintenance allowance for lone-parent families, a proposal that was never implemented. Child benefit replaced family allowances in an attempt to improve its redistributive impact, both between and within families.

These developments reflected a changing climate of opinion, notably the emergence of feminism. From the late 1960s, the women's movement highlighted the changing role of women within and outside the family and challenged family policy through critiques of the family and the welfare state. Issues such as abortion, contraception, domestic violence, cohabitation, and childcare provision were added to the policy agenda (Pascall 1997). There were policy changes in response to women's growing employment, including equal pay and sex discrimination legislation, SERPS (State Earnings Related Pension Scheme) and employment benefits for working mothers, including maternity benefits and optional unpaid maternity leave.

This activity reached its zenith with the announcement of a 'national family policy' to reconcile the new role of women at work with their traditional role within the family:

> The family is the most important unit in our community. That is why for the first time in our country our government is putting forward a national family policy. Our aim is straightforward: it is to strengthen the stability and quality of family life in Britain ... to pay more attention to how industry organises women's role at

work, so that her influence as the centre of the family, and the woman is usually the centre of the family, is not weakened.

(Prime Minister James Callaghan in 1977, quoted in Kamerman and Kahn 1997, p. 95)

Financial crisis and political divisions then ripped apart Labour's 'social contract' offering (but not delivering) a 'social wage' through welfare benefits in return for wage moderation. The notorious 'winter of discontent' discredited Labour's corporatist approach and the post-war consensus ended with a decisive Conservative win in the 1979 election.

THE TORY YEARS: 1979–1997

We are the party of the family.

(Margaret Thatcher 1977, quoted in Henwood and Wicks 1988, p. 7)

The years after 1979 were a period of retrenchment in public expenditure and greater reliance on private and family provision, e.g. in home ownership, private health care and pensions and community care. The welfare state was cast less as a primary provider of services (increasingly the family's role), than as a safety net if family and market provision failed. The family emerged as a morally contested terrain, with each party vying to appropriate 'the family' and 'family values'. The Conservatives championed the traditional family against changes undermining 'British' family life of the earlier post-war years. As Margaret Thatcher stated, 'there is no such thing as society; only individuals and families'. Major added his own touch, launching the back-firing 'back to basics' campaign. There was increasing emphasis on the family as a private domain; a bastion of freedom and protector of liberty against encroachment by the state. To critics, this often seemed a thinly coded call for self-reliance by families to reduce dependency on a 'nanny state'.

Much was made of traditional family values, espousing the breadwinner father and homemaker mother, whose primary responsibility was at home, whether or not she chose to work. The home was the place to inculcate 'family values' such as personal responsibility, obligations to care, respect for authority and property, and the work ethic. Unless labour supply was tight, the decision of mothers whether to work was seen as a private lifestyle choice. Generally, childcare was seen as a private responsibility and state provision of childcare an unwarranted burden. Non-traditional families with children were increasingly deprecated as part of the 'dependency culture' and depicted in terms ranging from second best to deviant and a pathological threat to the moral order of society. Lone mothers, notably single mothers, were singled out as especially threatening – here was the breeding ground of 'the underclass'. This period witnessed a succession of moral panics about the 'crisis' of the British family.

But this was also a period of major demographic change and labour market restructuring. Male unemployment rates rose dramatically, standing at 14% in 1993 (Hills 1998, p. 5). Marriage declined as the defining institution of the family, increasingly replaced by parenthood and children. A new focus emerged on child protection, notably in the Children Act 1989 and the Children (Scotland) Act 1995. Family policies became increasingly centred around children. Whatever the conference rhetoric, the government could bend to the breeze. Thus, to reduce the financial and social costs of family conflict, the Family Law Act 1996 removed the fault-based grounds for divorce and extended protection from domestic violence to cohabitees.

Despite this pragmatist undercurrent, the New Right agenda had a substantial impact. Child Benefit barely survived the retreat from universalism and horizontal redistribution. A greater emphasis on selectivity, targeting and means-testing was evident in changes initiated by the Social Security Act 1986 and the planned reduction in benefits to lone-parent families (although interrupted by the 1997 election and implemented by the incoming Labour government). Family policies were increasingly directed at problem families or families in need. Meanwhile the boundaries of family responsibility were extended both up and down the generations (through benefit reductions for young adults and community care for older people) and also into new family forms. Thus the Child Support Act 1991 reduced state support for lone-parent families, and shifted the burden towards 'absent' fathers.

During this period, the European Union's role in family policy became more significant. The European Parliament resolved in 1983 to 'identify and take into account those aspects of Community economic, social and cultural policy which relate to the family', to 'promote the launching of family policies in the member states' (Gauthier 1996, p. 149). The EU challenged British failures to help families reconcile work and family life or enhance the limited range of benefits to families; challenges often resisted by the UK government.

At the close of this era, British family policy was characterized by Kamerman and Kahn (1997, pp. 25–26) as 'modest and reluctant'. The Conservative governments left a legacy of greater inequality between families and child poverty within them. The poorest families did not share in the growing prosperity of the country. One estimate suggests that one child in three (4.3 million) is now living in a family with an income below half the national average. The comparable figure for 1968 was one in ten.

NEW LABOUR

In 1997, a Labour government was elected with a modernizing agenda, not only for welfare but for all areas of British life. But inertia is a powerful force in government. It is too early to judge how far policies will be changed by the Labour government. Will privatization be reversed and state provision increased? Will the trend towards greater targeting continue? How will the boundaries between state and family be redrawn? Will Britain's resistance to EU policy relax? Will Britain adopt a more continental European approach to family policy and social provision generally? Will ideas about family responsibility change?

Building on the past

The roots of New Labour can be found in the long social democratic tradition influencing the Labour movement of the twentieth century, including Fabian socialism and Christian or ethical humanism. These held that socialism, as a form of collectivism, could coexist with a capitalist state. The state, with its expert administrators, could become a vehicle for social reform to remedy social ills and achieve a fairer society. Its concept of citizenship emphasized duties more than rights – and with it, the idea of citizen participation. It embraced social rights of citizenship, but stressed equality of status and opportunity, rather than equality of outcomes.

New Labour has reaffirmed the idea of citizenship more as a set of duties than rights:

> A decent society is not based on rights. It is based on duty. Our duty to each other. To all should be given opportunity, from all responsibility demanded.
>
> (Tony Blair in 1997, quoted in Lister 1998, p. 222)

> Our reform agenda is dominated by a new emphasis on responsibilities as well as rights: the responsibility of parents, absent and present, to care, emotionally and materially for their children; the responsibility of adults of working age to work; the responsibility of welfare recipients to take opportunities to escape from dependency.
>
> (Minister for Welfare Reform in 1997, quoted in Lister 1998, p. 222).

Labour's current stress on the fulfilment of duties as a hallmark (and condition) of citizenship reflects the impact of New Right discourse on the underclass and dependency, although it does not represent a marked departure from earlier traditions.

The Labour government took office with some grand ambitions for the overhaul of welfare, notably in plans to develop alternative forms of collective social support. More recently, there has been greater stress on individual responsibilities and selective support, through more extensive means-testing of benefits. Labour's agenda tends to focus on limited redistribution to the poor:

> I believe in greater equality. If the next Labour Government has not raised the living standards of the poorest by the end of its term in office, it will have failed.
>
> (Tony Blair in 1996, quoted in Hills 1998, p. 29)

Thus Labour's egalitarian ambitions have narrowed to reducing poverty and social exclusion, the latter largely conceived in terms of exclusion from employment.

Family policy

Labour's family policy agenda favours a pragmatic approach, more tolerant of family diversity and going with the grain of social and economic change. This was evident in *The Family Way,* a family policy blueprint published by IPPR (the Labour think tank) in 1990, and written by Anna Coote, Harriet Harman and Patricia Hewitt – the last two becoming government ministers after 1997. It was evident too in *Supporting Families* (Home Office/Ministerial Group on the Family 1998), which aimed to 'swim with the tide' of change and preferred a piecemeal, practical approach, through better information, education and mediation, to improve people's capacities for parenting or managing relationship conflicts. New Labour still endorsed the 'first among equals' philosophy that privileges one family form – marriage – as the 'surest foundation' of the family. But even New Labour's pro-marriage polemic proffered only rather low-key pragmatic proposals, including a new role for registrars to give prenuptial counselling, prenuptial agreements, marriage preparation packs and baby naming ceremonies.

New Labour's modernizing agenda apparently recognizes that reinstating the traditional family can no longer be a goal of family policy. Anthony Giddens makes this point in his influential book, *The Third Way*:

> Take the family, which figures in some of the most contentious debates in modern politics. Sustaining continuity in family life, especially protecting the well-being of children, is one of the most important goals of family policy. This can't be achieved, however, through a reactionary stance, an attempt to reinstate the "traditional family" ... It presumes a modernising agenda of democratisation.
>
> (Giddens 1998, p. 68)

Giddens argues that 'third way' politics requires a new politics of the family:

> Family policy is a key test for the new politics: is there a politics of the family beyond neoliberalism and old-style social democracy?
>
> (Giddens 1998, p. 89)

A return to the traditional family is rejected on the grounds that:

- It is a nostalgic fantasy.
- Modern marriage has become a more egalitarian relationship, based on love and emotional attachment.
- Reproduction is no longer the primary rationale for marriage; childhood and child rearing have changed.
- Reversing demographic and economic change of this order is beyond the power of political institutions.

However, complete acceptance of growing diversity is also rejected, given the disadvantages associated with divorce and lone-parent families. For Giddens (1998, p. 95), the alternative is 'the democratic family', which involves:

- emotional and sexual equality
- mutual rights and responsibilities in relationships
- co-parenting
- life-long parental contracts
- negotiated authority over children
- obligations of children to parents
- the socially-integrated family.

The stress on parenthood rather than partnership reflects a focus on children:

> The protection and care of children is the single most important thread that should guide family policy
>
> (Giddens 1998, p. 94)

Family policies to promote this agenda include equal rights and responsibilities for fathers (irrespective of marital status or residence) and making parental commitment to a child contractual.

While these ideas break with Conservative thinking about the family (itself changing under new leadership) there is nevertheless considerable continuity. Selectivity and targeting seem set to continue, with no significant move (child benefit increases aside) towards greater universalism. So too are internal or quasi-markets in social provision. The language of public/private partnership persists, along with mixed forms of provision in social care and pensions. However, this no longer sanctifies the market so enthusiastically, being couched more in terms of social inclusion and social justice.

Social inclusion and social exclusion

Levitas (quoted by Lister 1998, p. 221) has identified three discourses on social inclusion and exclusion. The first emphasizes citizenship and social rights, with social justice as its main objective. The second emphasizes individual behaviour and values, and aims to reduce dependency. The third emphasizes exclusion from paid work, with social cohesion as its main objective. It is this last discourse that may best describe the New Labour approach. But elements of the other discourses also inform Labour policies. Although the 1999 budget provided gains to all income groups, those at the top gained only marginally, with those at the bottom (the poorest 30% and especially the poorest 10%) gaining most. This suggests that New Labour is committed to some measure of vertical redistribution, even if this is not part of Labour's current vocabulary. Even the Treasury has made a commitment to reducing inequality and poverty. This redistributive agenda has its limits, since it remains covert and largely focused on poverty rather than inequality.

New Labour has also embraced a moralistic discourse, most evident in measures to allow curfews on young children, to oblige parents to monitor homework and to hold parents responsible for young offenders; but also apparent in proposals to tackle the so-called 'dependency' culture, notably the threat to withdraw benefits from lone parents not attending regular interviews intended to get them back to work. As was argued in relation to financial obligations of non-resident parents, 'personal circumstances cannot negate responsibility' even for those on benefit.

Welfare reform

The 'big idea' behind Labour's welfare reforms has the (paid) work ethic at its core. This is seen as the best means to achieve economic security and social inclusion. The decision to implement planned Conservative cuts in lone-parent benefits expressed a resolve to make work rewarding, even by penalizing families entirely reliant on benefit. The welfare to work reforms have revolved around various New Deals targeted at different groups in order to increase their labour market participation. A variety of other measures are designed to 'make work pay', notably the Working Families Tax Credit, the new Childcare Tax Credit, the 10p income tax band and the National Minimum Wage. Other measures include the reform of child support, the National Childcare Strategy, and the National Carers Strategy. See Figure 7.1 for a summary of Labour policies relevant to family policy.

New Labour has changed the parameters of debate. Whether these initiatives will realize their promise is another matter. For example, the proposed Working Families Tax Credit has been variously criticized as liable to encourage fraud, penalize lone parents, redistribute resources away from mothers, and (contrary to its intention) create disincentives to work. But even such an apparently innocuous policy as Labour's new homework guidelines may prove counter-productive, given evidence suggesting that extra homework may not raise educational standards, as moderate amounts of homework may be better than a little or a lot. Labour's emphasis on more education and advice as a remedy for social problems such as divorce looks less persuasive with the failure of the advisory and mediation services established following the 1996 Family Law Act. The advisory service when piloted failed to reach more than one in ten divorcing couples; and of these, very few accepted referral to mediation or counselling. Those attending mediation were more not less likely to see a solicitor following advice received. Since

Figure 7.1. Summary of government policies since May 1997 relevant to family policy

- *Supporting Families* Green Paper (Home Office/Ministerial Group on the Family 1998).
- *New ambitions for our country: a new contract for welfare,* the 1998 DSS welfare reform Green Paper, including various New Deals such as those for lone parents, the long-term unemployed and partners of unemployed people.
- Working Families Tax Credit (and the Childcare Tax Credit), (*Supporting Families,* Home Office/Ministerial Group on the Family 1998).
- *Children First,* Green Paper with proposals for reforming child support (DSS 1998).
- *A new contract for welfare: Children's Rights and Parents' Responsibilities:* (DSS 1999). The White Paper plans to reform the child support system.
- National insurance reformed.
- Budget increases in Child Benefit (April 1999 and April 2000).
- National Childcare Strategy, DfEE/DSS 1998 Green Paper.
- National Minimum Wage, introduced in 1999 by the DTI.
- National Carers Strategy in *Caring about Carers,* Department of Health 1999 White Paper.
- *No More Excuses,* Home Office 1997 Green Paper with proposals on parental responsibility for children's behaviour.
- Lord Chancellor's Department 1998 Green Paper on parental responsibility for unmarried fathers.
- *Fairness at Work,* DTI White Paper in 1998, to implement EU initiatives on reconciling work and family life into UK policy, including the EU Parental Leave Directive, EU Working Time Directive and the EU Part-Time Work Directive.

the advisory service has proved ineffectual and perhaps even counter-productive, the government has shelved plans to extend it nation-wide. So much for a measure intended to reduce divorce or mitigate the conflicts attending it.

Family policy

Will such policies promote greater consensus about family life and how society should support families? Do these amount to a

UK family policy? This is a story that is still being written. There are moves towards a more explicit national family policy. But will they constitute a sufficiently integrated and comprehensive package? Coherence in policy formulation and implementation requires more than policy change; it needs changes to the structure, machinery and composition of government. With greater representation of women in Parliament, family policy may (or may not) receive greater political priority. There has been more focus at Cabinet level on family issues since the setting up of the Women's Unit and the Social Exclusion Unit in the Cabinet Office in 1997. Labour's programme of devolution also offers an opportunity to bring government 'closer to the people' and democratize policy-making processes that most affect the family.

Nevertheless, Labour's approach tends to be pragmatic, piecemeal and long-term, wary of major reforms and large-scale commitments. Its cool reception of the Royal Commission's recommendation that personal care for older people should be funded through taxation casts doubt on the prospects for a more comprehensive and integrated approach. Gauthier's speculation about the future of family policy in an international context seems to apply to Britain.

> State support for families is likely to remain a major political issue during the next decades, but budget constraints will severely limit government action. In particular, the issues of targeting of cash benefits, reconciliation between employment and family responsibilities, and employers' involvement are likely to characterize future trends in family policy.
>
> (Gauthier 1996, p. 207)

Any attempt to restructure family policy is bound to face difficulties. Family policy does not deal with specific forms of state provision of goods, money or services. It is not defined by a function or specific activity of government, as is health, social security or education. Thus family policy is not institutionalized. There is no structure in government to correspond to family policy (e.g. a Department of the Family) and no minister of the family whose remit covers the full range of family policies. Despite the first efforts of the Ministerial Group on the Family, family policy is still dispersed across government departments in its formulation and implementation. There is still no requirement that social and public policies should be evaluated in terms of their effects on families; still no 'family impact' statements for public policies which would consider the likely implications of policies for families; and still no requirement that family policies should be assessed as a whole for consistency and comprehensiveness.

Despite this, it seems unreasonable to claim, as Kamerman and Kahn (1978) once did, that Britain has no family policy. Policies that implicitly influence family life and well-being have a long tradition. Ringen and colleagues (Kamerman and Kahn 1997, p. 97) suggest that there is a form of 'reluctant' family policy in Britain, whereby policies are brought forward by government if:

- 'they identify *problems* in the family, either in performing what are seen as family functions in society or with respect to internal pressures and strains in families'
- 'pressures for government intervention are not overridden by what are considered to be *constraints* on the scope of government action'
- 'they believe it is in their power to intervene effectively with respect to the problems that are identified.' [their italics]

Despite the ideological battles over 'family values' in the 1990s, this approach – oriented to problems, limited by constraints and focused on effectiveness – still seems likely to form the general framework within which family policy evolves in Britain.

KEY POINTS

- The British approach to family policy has been implicit and non-interventionist, with selective intervention based on need and 'problem families'. In the early twentieth century, family policy limited state intervention to where serious problems or needs existed in 'problem families'. Family policy in the post-war era is divided into three periods: the post-war consensus, the Conservative era from 1979 and the post-1997 Labour period.
- The Beveridge Report introduced limited universalism in social security provisions for all families, assuming a breadwinner model of the family, full male employment, economically inactive wives and lifelong marriage. Social and economic change made these assumptions increasingly incorrect.
- The Conservative period from 1979 introduced a New Right agenda with more reliance on private and family provision. Family policies emphasized selectivity, targeting and means-testing, centred on children and problem families, and saw the

welfare state as a safety net against market or family failure. Married women's growing economic activity and the growth in divorce and lone parenthood fuelled debates about the 'crisis' in the family.

- New Labour's modernizing agenda emphasizes equality of opportunity, citizenship defined more by responsibilities than rights, a strong (paid) work ethic and reducing child poverty and social exclusion. The family policy agenda is a pragmatic 'third way', more tolerant of family diversity with more emphasis on parenthood than partnership. A more explicit family policy is emerging, with a larger state role in supporting families.

GUIDE TO FURTHER READING

For a review of family policies before 1997, see:

Kamerman, S. B. and Kahn, A. J. (eds) (1997) *Family change and family policies in Great Britain, Canada, New Zealand, and the United States,* Oxford: Clarendon Press, pp. 31–100 especially pp. 92–100 about the politics of family policy.

For an assessment of the period 1979–1997, see:

Hills, J. (1998) *Thatcherism, New Labour and the Welfare State,* London: CASE/LSE.

Lister, R. (1996) 'Back to the family: Family policy and politics under the Major government' in Millar, J. and Jones, H. (eds) (1996) *The Politics of the Family,* London: Avebury, pp. 11–31.

For a view of where family policy fits in the 'third way' of New Labour thinking, see:

Giddens, A. (1998) *The Third Way: the renewal of social democracy,* Cambridge: Polity Press, Chapter 3.

For an early assessment of family policies since 1997, see:

Lister, R. (1998) 'From equality to social inclusion: New Labour and the welfare state' *Critical Social Policy 55,* pp. 215–225.

Useful websites

Family policy is an area of study in which up-to-date information is particularly important. Many of the documents that we refer to in this book are available in full or in summary form over the internet. Policy documents can appear on the web sooner than in printed form. When searching for information on the internet, it is more efficient to have some useful starting points to focus your search.

Information gateways

SOSIG *http://www.sosig.ac.uk/*
The Social Science Information Gateway (SOSIG) provides academic researchers and practitioners with access to networked information resources worldwide.

CCTA Government Information Service *http://www.open.gov.uk/*
CCTA (Central Computer and Telecommunications Agency) is a starting point for web links to a wide range of central and local government websites.

BOPCAS *http://www.soton.ac.uk/~bopcas/*
BOPCAS (British Official Publications Current Awareness Service) is a database of UK official publications, which you can search for government publications, including HMSO publications. It includes Acts of Parliament, Command Papers, Departmental Publications, Green Papers, House of Commons Bills, Papers, Library Research Papers and House of Lords Bills and Papers.

Information and documents from government departments

The home pages of government departments often have links to recent policy documents and press releases. Here are a few websites (which you can also access via CCTA).

The Treasury *http://www.hm-treasury.gov.uk/*

Department of Social Security *http://www.dss.gov.uk/*

The Department of Health *http://www.doh.gov.uk*

The Home Office *http://www.homeoffice.gov.uk*

Other internet sources for information and research on family policy

The Family Policy Studies Centre has a very useful website with lots of up-to-date information and research on family policy.
Family Policy Studies Centre *http://www.vois.org.uk/fpsc/*

The Joseph Rowntree Foundation publishes abbreviated research findings relevant to family policy in its Findings series, available at its website:
Joseph Rowntree Foundation *http://www.jrf.org.uk/*

Policy documents on the web

The government publishes many consultation documents on the internet (although they tend to be removed after a while). Most can be downloaded. At the time of writing, the following documents were accessible on the web.

Welfare Reform Green Paper, 1998, *New Ambitions for our country: a new contract for welfare,* Department of Social Security, March 1998, Cm 3805.
http://www.dss.gov.uk/hq/wreform/mainframe.htm

Home Office/Ministerial Group on the Family, 1998, *Supporting Families.*
http://www.homeoffice.gov.uk/vcu/sfpages.pdf

CHAPTER 2

For some demographic snapshots of Britain, see the website of Office for National Statistics *http://www.ons.gov.uk/*

At the Home Office website, see the Ministerial Group on the Family 1998 Consultation Paper *Supporting Families* (see Chapter 1).

See the Joseph Rowntree Foundation website for a summary of *'Private lives and public responses: lone parenthood and future policy',* by Ford, R. and Millar, J. (1997) Joseph Rowntree Foundation Foundations, July.

CHAPTER 3

The government view on parental responsibility for the behaviour of children can be seen in two Home Office documents: *No more excuses* (1997) and *Supporting Families* (1998) (see Chapter 1).

CHAPTER 4

Community care

Royal Commission on Long Term Care:
http://www.officialdocuments.co.uk/document/cm41/4192/4192.htm

Department of Health 1999 White Paper, *Caring about Carers* (The National Strategy for Carers)
http://www.doh.gov.uk/pub/docs/doh/care.pdf

On domestic violence

The Home Office domestic violence website
http://www.homeoffice.gov.uk/cpd/cpsu/domviol98.htm#1

The Lord Chancellor's Department guide to the domestic violence provisions of the Family Law Act 1996
http://www.open.gov.uk/lcd/family/dvguidfr.htm

Domestic violence data source website with links to other information.
http://www.domesticviolencedata.org/

Women's Aid Federation England website
http://www.womensaid.org.uk/

CHAPTER 5

Data about low-income households can be found in

Department of Social Security (1998): *Households Below Average Income 1979 to 1996/7*, (HBAI), London: The Stationery Office:
http://www.dss.gov.uk/asd/hbai/hbai98.html

The Welfare Reform Green Paper is at
http://www.dss.gov.uk/hq/wreform/mainframe.htm

Information about the Working Families Tax Credit (WFTC) can be found at the Treasury website at
http://www.hm-treasury.gov.uk/pub/html/budget98/wftc.pdf

The 1999 Child Support White Paper (*A new contract for welfare: Children's Rights and Parents' Responsibilities*, Cm 4349) is at *http://www.dss.gov.uk/hq/pubs/childsup/index.htm*

CHAPTER 6

Home Office (1998) *Supporting Families* (Ministerial Group on the Family) website:
http://www.homeoffice.gov.uk/vcu/sfpages.pdf

National Childcare Strategy Green Paper, May 1998, (*Meeting the Childcare Challenge*), Departments of Education and Employment and the Department of Social Security
http://www.open.gov.uk/dfee/childcare/

Department of Trade and Industry White Paper (1998) *Fairness at Work*. See Chapter 5 on family-friendly policies.
http://www.dti.gov.uk/IR/fairness/part5.htm

List of references

Arendell, T. (1995) *Fathers and Divorce,* London: Sage.

Backett, K. C. (1982) *Mothers and fathers: a study of the development and negotiation of parental behaviour,* London: Macmillan.

Baldock, J. (1993) 'Old age' in Dallos, R. and McLaughlin, E. (eds) (1993) *Social Problems and the Family,* London: Sage.

Berthoud, R. and Ford, R. (1996) *A new way of measuring relative financial needs, Joseph Rowntree Foundation Findings Social Policy Research 109,* York: Joseph Rowntree Foundation.

Beveridge, W. H. (1942) *Report of the Interdepartmental Committee on Social Insurance and Allied Services (The Beveridge Report),* London: HMSO.

Bradshaw, J. and Stimson, C. (1997) *Using Child Benefit in the Family Budget,* London: The Stationery Office/SPRU.

Brannen, J., Mezaros, G., Moss, P. and Polan, G. (1994) *Employment and Family Life: A review of research in the UK, Research Series No. 41,* London: Department of Employment.

Brown, C. (1999) 'Middle class loses out as children gain', *The Independent* 10 March 1999.

Bryson, A. and Marsh, A. (1996) *Leaving family credit: a survey carried out on behalf of the Department of Social Security by the Policy Studies Institute: Department of Social Security Research Report No. 48,* London: HMSO.

Burgess, A. and Ruxton, S. (1998) 'Men and their children' in Franklin, J. (ed.) (1998) *Social Policy and Social Justice,* Cambridge: Polity.

Burghes, L. (1994) *Lone parenthood and family disruption: the outcomes for children,* London: Family Policy Studies Centre.

Burghes, L. and Brown, M. (1995) *Single Lone Mothers: Problems, Prospects and Policies,* London: Family Policy Studies Centre.

Burghes, L., Clarke, L. and Cronin, N. (1997) *Fathers and fatherhood in Britain,* London: Family Policy Studies Centre.

Cabinet Office (1998) *Tackling domestic violence,* London: Cabinet Office.

Callender, C. (1996) 'Women and employment' in Hallett, C. (ed.) (1996) *Women and Social Policy: an introduction,* Hemel Hempstead: Harvester Wheatsheaf.

Clarke, K., Glendinning, C. and Craig, G. (1994) *Losing Support: Children and the Child Support Act,* London: The Children's Society.

Clarke, L. (1996) 'Demographic change and the family situation of children' in Brannen, J. and O'Brien, M. (eds) (1996) *Children in Families: Research and Policy*, London: Falmer Press.

Cockett, M. and Tripp, J. (1994) *Children living in re-ordered families, Joseph Rowntree Foundation Findings No. 45*, York: Joseph Rowntree Foundation.

Cohen, D. (1997) 'Five steps to married bliss', *The Independent* 26 February 1997.

Cohen, B. and Fraser, N. (1991) *Childcare in a Modern Welfare System*, London: IPPR.

Coles, B. (1998) 'Young people' in Alcock, P., Erskine, A. and May, M. (eds) (1998) *The Student's Companion to Social Policy*, Oxford: Blackwell and the Social Policy Association.

Cooper, G. (1997) 'Couples unable to adopt gain right to appeal', *The Independent* 18 February 1997.

Cooper, G. (1998) 'Male nurses leave women in slow lane', *The Independent* 6 August 1998.

Coote, A. (1995) 'The family: a battleground in fearful times', *The Independent* 30 October 1995.

Coote, A., Harman, H. and Hewitt, P. (1990) *The Family Way*, London: IPPR.

Coote, A., Harman, H. and Hewitt, P. (1998) 'Family Policy: Guidelines and Goals' in Franklin, J. (ed.) (1998) *Social Policy and Social Justice*, Cambridge: Polity Press (with IPPR).

Craven, E., Rimmer, L. and Wicks, M. (1982) *Family issues and public policy*, London: Study Commission on the Family.

Dallos, R. and McLaughlin, E. (eds) (1993) *Social Problems and the Family*, London: Sage.

Daniel, P. and Ivatts, J. (1998) *Children and Social Policy*, Basingstoke, Macmillan.

Dean, H. (1997) 'Underclassed or undermined? Young people and social citizenship' in MacDonald, R. (ed.) (1997) *Youth, the Underclass and Social Exclusion*, London: Routledge.

Dench, G. (1996) *Exploring variations in men's family roles Joseph Rowntree Foundation Findings No. 99*, York: Joseph Rowntree Foundation.

Dennis, N. and Erdos, G. (1993) *Families without Fatherhood* (Second edition), London: IEA (Institute for Economic Affairs Health and Welfare Unit).

Department for Education and Employment and the Department of Social Security (1998) *Meeting the Childcare Challenge: a framework and consultation document (National Childcare Strategy Green Paper)*, Cm 3959.

Department of Health (1998) *Working Together to Safeguard Children: New Government Proposals for Inter-agency Co-operation*, London: Department of Health.

Department of Health (1999) *White Paper: Caring about Carers, (The National Strategy for Carers)*, London: The Stationery Office.

Department of Social Security (1998a) *Households Below Average Income 1979 to 1996/7, (HBAI)*, London: The Stationery Office.

Department of Social Security (1998b) *Welfare reform focus file 7: children and families.*

Department of Social Security (1998c) *Children First: a new approach to child support*, Cm 3992, London: The Stationery Office.

Department of Social Security (1998d) *Welfare Reform Green Paper, New Ambitions for our country: a new contract for welfare*, March 1998, Cm 3805 (Welfare Reform Green Paper).

Department of Social Security (1999) *Child Support White Paper: A new contract for welfare: Children's Rights and Parents' Responsibilities*, CM 4349, London: DSS.

Department of Trade and Industry (1998) *White Paper Fairness at Work*, Cm 3968, London: DTI.

Dickens, R., Fry, V. and Pashardes, P. (1995) *The cost of children and the welfare state, Joseph Rowntree Foundation Findings No. 89*, York: Joseph Rowntree Foundation.

Dobash, R. E. and Dobash, R. P. (1979) *Violence Against Wives: a case against the patriarchy*, New York: Free Press.

Dobash, R. E. and Dobash, R. P. (1992) *Women, Violence and Social Change*, London: Routledge.

Dobson, R. and Moyes, J. (1996) 'What makes marriage heaven or hell', *The Independent* 2 August 1996

Dowler, E. and Calvert, C. (1995) *Nutrition and diet in lone-parent families in London*, London : Family Policy Studies Centre.

Edwards, L. and Griffiths, A. (1997) *Family Law*, Edinburgh: W. Green/Sweet and Maxwell.

Edwards, R. and Duncan, S. (1996) 'Rational economic man or lone mothers in context? the uptake of paid work' Chapter 6 in Silva, E. B. (ed.) (1996) *Good Enough Mothering: Feminist perspectives on lone mothering*, London: Routledge.

Ermisch, J. (1997) *Family Matters*, Essex: Centre for Economic Policy Research.

Family Policy Studies Centre (1998a) 'Families and money', *Family Policy Bulletin*, Autumn, London: FPSC.

Family Policy Studies Centre (1998b) 'Families and childcare', *Family Briefing Paper 6*, London: FPSC.

Ferri, E. and Smith, K. (1996) *Parenting in the 1990s*, London: Family Policy Studies Centre.

Ferriman, A. (1997) 'Sex harassment rife in mental hospital wards', *The Independent* 4 March 1997

Finch, J. and Mason, J. (1993) *Negotiating Family Responsibilities*, London: Tavistock/Routledge.

Ford, R., Marsh, A. and McKay, S. (1995) *Changes in Lone Parenthood*, London: HMSO.

Gano-Phillips, S. and Fincham, F. D. (1995) 'Family conflict, divorce and children's adjustment' in Fitzpatrick, M. A. and Vangelisti, A. L. (eds) (1995) *Explaining Family Interactions*, London: Sage.

Gauthier, A. H. (1996) *The State and the Family: a Comparative Analysis of Family Policies in Industrialized Countries*, Oxford: Clarendon Press.

Giddens, A. (1998) *The Third Way: the renewal of social democracy*, Cambridge: Polity Press.

Goode, J., Callender, C. and Lister, R. (1998) *Purse or Wallet?* London: Policy Studies Institute.

Goodnow, J. J. and Bowes, J. M. (1994) *Men, women and household work*, Oxford: Oxford University Press.

Grice, A. (1999) 'Ministers to take hard line on single mothers', *The Independent* 10 February 1999.

Hantrais, L. (1999) 'Comparing family policies in Europe' in Clasen, J. (ed.) (1999) *Comparative Social Policy*, Oxford: Blackwell.

Hantrais, L. and Letablier, M. (1996) *Families and Family Policies in Europe*, London: Longman.

Harding, L. F. (1996) *Family, State and Social Policy*, Basingstoke: Macmillan.

Harker, L. (1996) *A secure future? Social security and the family in a changing world*, London: Child Poverty Action Group.

Harkness, S., Machin, S. and Waldfogel, J. (1994) *Women's pay and family income inequality, Joseph Rowntree Foundation Findings No. 60*, York: Joseph Rowntree Foundation.

Haskey, J. (1998) in David, M. E. (ed.) (1998) *The Fragmenting Family: does it matter?*, London: IEA (Institute for Economic Affairs Health and Welfare Unit).

Henwood, M. and Wicks, M. (1986) *Benefit or Burden? The objectives and impact of child support*, London: Family Policy Studies Centre.

Hewitt, P. (1993) *About Time: The revolution in work and family life*, London: Rivers Oram Press.

Hill, M. and Aldgate, J. (1996) 'The Children Act 1989 and recent developments in research in England and Wales' in Hill, M. and Aldgate, J. (eds) (1996) *Child Welfare Services: Developments in law, policy, practice and research*, London: Jessica Kingsley.

Hill, M. and Aldgate, J. (eds) (1996) Child Welfare Services: *Developments in law, policy, practice and research*, London: Jessica Kingsley.

Hills, J. (1998) *Thatcherism, New Labour and the Welfare State*, London: CASE/LSE.

HM Treasury (1998) *The Modernisation of Britain's Tax and Benefit System Number Three: The Working Families Tax Credit and work incentives*, London: HM Treasury.

HM Treasury (1999) *Tackling Poverty and Extending Opportunity: the modernisation of Britain's tax and benefit system number four*, London: HM Treasury.

Home Office (1997) *No more excuses: a new approach to tackling youth crime in England and Wales*, London: The Stationery Office.

Home Office Criminal Policy Strategy Unit (1999) *Domestic Violence*, London: Home Office, http://www.homeoffice.gov.uk/cpd/cpsu/domviol98.htm#1.

Home Office/Ministerial Group on the Family (1998) *Supporting Families*, London: Home Office and Voluntary and Community Unit.

Jacques, M. (1996) 'Decline and fallacy', *The Guardian* 9 November 1996

Jones, G. (1995) *Leaving home*, Buckingham: Open University Press.

Jones, G. and Wallace, C. (1992) *Youth, Family and Citizenship*, Buckingham: Open University Press.

Jones, S. (1993) *The Language of the Genes*, London: Flamingo.

Jordan, B., Jaes, S., Kay, H. and Redley, M. (1992) *Trapped in Poverty*, London: Routledge

Jordan, B., Redley, M. and James, S. (1994) *Putting the Family First: Identities, decisions, citizenship*, London: UCL Press.

Joshi, H., Ward, C., Dale, A. and Davies, H. (1995) *Dependence and independence in the finances of women aged 33*, London: Family Policy Studies Centre.

Judd, J. (1997) 'Labour tells parents: read to your children' *The Independent* 28 February 1997.

Jury, L. and Burrell, I. (1999) 'Mothers urged to give up babies' *The Independent* 26 January 1999.

Kamerman, S. B. and Kahn, A. J. (eds) (1978) Family Policy: *Government and Families in Fourteen Countries*, New York: Columbia University Press.

Kamerman, S. B. and Kahn, A. J. (eds) (1997) *Family change and family policies in Great Britain, Canada, New Zealand, and the United States*, Oxford: Clarendon Press.

Kempson, E. (1996) *Life on a Low Income*, London: Child Poverty Action Group.

Kiernan, K. E. (1995) *Transitions to parenthood: young mothers, young fathers – Associated factors and later life experiences: Discussion Paper 113*, London: Welfare State Programme Suntory-Toyota International Centre for Economics and Related Disciplines, London School of Economics.

Kiernan, K. E. (1997) *The legacy of parental divorce: social, economic and demographic experiences in adulthood*, London: London School of Economics and Political Science/Centre for Analysis of Social Exclusion.

Kiernan, K. (1998) in David, M. E. (ed.) (1998) *The Fragmenting Family: does it matter?*, London: IEA (Institute for Economic Affairs Health and Welfare Unit).

Kiernan, K. and Estaugh, V. (1993) *Cohabitation, Extra-marital Childbearing and Social Policy,* London: Policy Studies Institute.

Land, H. (1996) 'The Crumbling Bridges between Childhood and Adulthood' in Brannen, J. and O'Brien, M. (eds) (1996) *Children in Families: Research and Policy,* London: Falmer Press.

Lasch, C. (1977) *Haven in a heartless world: the family besieged,* New York: Basic Books.

Lewis, J. and Maclean, M. (1997) 'Recent developments in Family Policy in the UK: the case of the 1996 Family Law Act' in May, M., Brunsdon, E. and Craig, G. (eds) (1997) *Social Policy Review 9,* London: Social Policy Association.

Lister, R. (ed.) (1996) *Charles Murray and the Underclass: the developing debate,* London: Institute for Economic Affairs Health and Welfare Unit.

Lister, R. (1998) 'From equality to social inclusion: New Labour and the welfare state' *Critical Social Policy 55,* pp. 215–225.

MacDonald, R. (1997) *Youth, the 'Underclass' and Social Exclusion,* London: Routledge.

Maclean, M. and Kuh, D. (1991) 'The long term effect for girls of parental divorce' in Maclean, M. and Groves, D. (eds) (1991) *Women's Issues in Social Policy,* London: Routledge.

McRae, S. (1991) 'Occupational Change over Childbirth: evidence from a National Survey' *Sociology,* Nov, 25, 4, pp. 589–605.

McRae, S. (1993) *Cohabiting mothers: changing marriage and motherhood?* London: Policy Studies Institute.

Middleton, S., Ashworth, K. and Braithwaite, I. (1997) *Small Fortunes: Spending on children, childhood poverty and parental sacrifice,* York: Joseph Rowntree Foundation.

Millar, J. (1998) 'Social policy and family policy' in Alcock, P., Erskine, A. and May, M. (eds) (1998) *The Student's Companion to Social Policy,* Oxford: Blackwell and the Social Policy Association.

Morgan, P. (1995) *Farewell to the Family? Public Policy and Family Breakdown in Britain and the USA,* London: IEA (Institute for Economic Affairs Health and Welfare Unit).

Morgan, P. (1998) 'An endangered species?' in David, M. E. (ed.) (1998) *The Fragmenting Family: does it matter?,* London: IEA (Institute for Economic Affairs Health and Welfare Unit), pp. 65–82.

Morley, R. and Mullender, A. (1994) *Preventing Domestic Violence to Women,* Home Office CPU Paper 48, London: Home Office.

Morrow, V. and Richards, M. (1996) *Transitions to adulthood: A family matter?* York: Joseph Rowntree Foundation.

Moyes, J. (1997) 'Lesson one: Girls want to have sex', *The Independent* 25 February 1997.

Murphy, E. (1999) 'Children of 10 call for help on pregnancy' *The Independent* 25 March 1999.

Murray, C. (1994) *Underclass: the Crisis Deepens*, London: IEA (Institute for Economic Affairs Health and Welfare Unit).

Murray, C. (1999) *The Underclass Revisited* published by the American Enterprise Institute on the web at http://www.aei.org/ps/psmurray.htm

Murray, C., Field, F., Brown, J. C., Walker, A. and Deakin, N. (1990) *The Emerging British Underclass*, London: IEA (Institute for Economic Affairs Health and Welfare Unit).

Norton, C. (1999) 'Concern over babies born to fathers beyond grave', *The Independent* 12 July 1999.

O'Sullivan, J. (1996) 'Back to school for Mum and Dad', *The Independent* 14 November 1996.

Office for National Statistics (1997) *Living in Britain: Preliminary results from the 1995 General Household Survey*, London: The Stationery Office.

Office for National Statistics (1998) *Living in Britain: Results from the 1996 General Household Survey*, London: The Stationery Office.

Office for National Statistics (1999) 'Marriages and divorces during 1996, and adoptions in 1997: England and Wales', *Population Trends 95*.

Oldfield, N. and Autumn, C. S. Y. (1993) *The Cost of a Child: Living Standards for the 1990s*, London: Child Poverty Action Group.

OPCS Social Survey Division (1996) *Living in Britain: Results from the 1994 General Household Survey*, London: HMSO.

Oppenheim, C. and Harker, L. (1996) *Poverty, the Facts* (Third edition), London: Child Poverty Action Group.

Pahl, J. (1984) 'The allocation of money within the household' in Freeman, M. (ed.) (1984) *The State, the Law and the Family*, London: Tavistock.

Pahl, J. (1989) *Money and Marriage*, London: Macmillan.

Papps, I. (1980) *For love or money? A preliminary economic analysis of marriage and the family*, London: Institute of Economic Affairs.

Pascall, G. (1997) Social Policy: *A New Feminist Analysis*, London: Routledge.

Phoenix, A. (1991) *Young Mothers?* Cambridge: Polity Press in association with Basil Blackwell.

Phoenix, A. (1996) 'Social constructions of lone motherhood: a case of competing discourses' in Silva, E. B. (ed.) (1996) *Good Enough Mothering: Feminist perspectives on lone mothering*, London: Routledge.

Pugh, G., De'Ath, E. and Smith, C. (1994) *Confident Parents, Confident Children: policy and practice in parent education and support*, London: National Children's Bureau.

Ridley, M. (1994) *The Red Queen: Sex and the evolution of human nature*, London: Penguin.

Robertson, A.F. (1991) *Beyond the Family: The Social Organization of Human Reproduction*, Cambridge: Polity Press.

Robinson, M. (1991) *Family Transformation Through Divorce and Remarriage: A Systematic Approach*, London: Routledge.

Rodgers, B. and Pryor, J. (1998) *Divorce and separation: the outcomes for children*, York: Joseph Rowntree Foundation.

Roseneil, S. and Mann, K. (1996) 'Unpalatable choices and inadequate families: lone mothers and the underclass debate' in Silva, E. B. (ed.) (1996) *Good Enough Mothering: Feminist perspectives on lone mothering*, London: Routledge.

Saraga, E. (1993) 'The Abuse of children' in Dallos, R. and McLaughlin, E. (eds) (1993) *Social Problems and the Family*, London: Sage.

Selman, P. and Glendinning, C. (1996) 'Teenage pregnancy: do social policies make a difference?' in Brannen, J. and O'Brien, M. (eds) (1996) *Children in Families*, London: Falmer.

Sevehuijsen, S. (1989) 'The politics of gender and child custody: the portrait on the wall' in Brannen, J., Hantrais, L., O'Brien, M. and Wilson, G. (eds) (1989) *Cross-national Studies of Household Resources after Divorce*, Birmingham: Aston University.

Silva, E. B. (1996) 'The transformation of mothering' in Silva, E. B. (ed.) (1996) *Good Enough Mothering: feminist perspectives on lone motherhood*, London: Routledge.

Speak, S., Cameron, S., Woods, R. and Gilroy, R. (1995) *Young single mothers: Barriers to independent living*, York: Joseph Rowntree Foundation.

Spencer, N. (1996) 'Reducing child health inequalities' in Bywaters, P. and McLeod, E. (eds) (1996) *Working for Equality in Health*, London: Routledge.

Sweeting, H. and West, P. (1996) *The relationship between family life and young people's lifestyles, Joseph Rowntree Foundation Findings No. 95*, York: Joseph Rowntree Foundation.

Tisdall, K. (1996) 'From the Social Work (Scotland) Act 1968 to the Children (Scotland) Act 1995: pressures for change', in Hill, M. and Aldgate, J. (eds) (1996) *Child Welfare Services: Developments in law, policy, practice and research*, London: Jessica Kingsley, pp. 24–39.

Tudge, C. (1995) *The Day Before Yesterday*, London: Pimlico.

Twigg, J. and Atkin, K. (1994) *Carers Perceived: Policy and Practice in Informal Care*, Buckingham: Open University Press.

Ungerson, C. (1987) *Policy is Personal: Sex, Gender and Informal Care*, London: Tavistock.

Utting, D. (1995) *Family and parenthood: supporting families, preventing breakdown: a guide to the debate*, York: Joseph Rowntree Foundation.

Van Dyck, J. (1995) *Manufacturing babies and public consent: debating the new reproductive technologies*, New York: New York University Press.

Vogler, C. (1994) 'Money in the household' in Anderson, M., Bechhofer, F. and Gershuny, J. (eds) (1994) *The Social and Political Economy of the Household*, Oxford: Oxford University Press.

Ward, L. (1997a) 'Children's achievements likely to mirror their parents', *The Independent* 1 March 1997.

Ward, L. (1997b) 'Carey angers teachers with call for marriage lessons in school', *The Independent* 11 April 1997.

Ward, C., Dale, A. and Joshi, H. (1996) 'Combining employment with childcare: an escape from dependence', *Journal of Social Policy* 25(2), pp. 223–224.

Warnock, M. (1984) Department of Health and Social Security, *Report of the Committee of Inquiry into Human Fertilisation and Embryology* (The Warnock Report), Cmnd. 9314, London: HMSO.

Willetts, D. (1993) *The Family,* W H Smith Contemporary Papers.

Wilson, G. (1987) 'Money : Patterns of Responsibility and Irresponsibility in Marriage' in Brannen, J. and Wilson, G. (eds) (1987) *Give and Take in Families: Studies in Resource Distribution,* London: Allen and Unwin.

Women's Aid Federation of England (1995) Annual Survey, pubished by WAFE on the web at http://www.womensaid.org.uk/stats/statuser.htm.

Women's Aid Federation of England (1996) Women's Aid briefing paper – August 1996, London: WAFE.

Zimmerman, S. L. (1995) *Understanding family policy: theories and applications,* Thousand Oaks, Calif.: Sage.

Index